The OECD Health Project

Towards High-Performing Health Systems

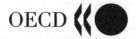
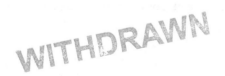
OECD

ORGANISATION FOR ECONOMIC CO-OPERATION AND DEVELOPMENT

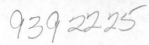

ORGANISATION FOR ECONOMIC CO-OPERATION AND DEVELOPMENT

Pursuant to Article 1 of the Convention signed in Paris on 14th December 1960, and which came into force on 30th September 1961, the Organisation for Economic Co-operation and Development (OECD) shall promote policies designed:

- to achieve the highest sustainable economic growth and employment and a rising standard of living in member countries, while maintaining financial stability, and thus to contribute to the development of the world economy;

- to contribute to sound economic expansion in member as well as non-member countries in the process of economic development; and

- to contribute to the expansion of world trade on a multilateral, non-discriminatory basis in accordance with international obligations.

The original member countries of the OECD are Austria, Belgium, Canada, Denmark, France, Germany, Greece, Iceland, Ireland, Italy, Luxembourg, the Netherlands, Norway, Portugal, Spain, Sweden, Switzerland, Turkey, the United Kingdom and the United States. The following countries became members subsequently through accession at the dates indicated hereafter: Japan (28th April 1964), Finland (28th January 1969), Australia (7th June 1971), New Zealand (29th May 1973), Mexico (18th May 1994), the Czech Republic (21st December 1995), Hungary (7th May 1996), Poland (22nd November 1996), Korea (12th December 1996) and the Slovak Republic (14th December 2000). The Commission of the European Communities takes part in the work of the OECD (Article 13 of the OECD Convention).

Publié en français sous le titre :
LE PROJET DE L'OCDE SUR LA SANTÉ
Vers des systèmes de santé plus performants

Foreword

The OECD initiated the Health Project in 2001 to address some of the key challenges policy makers face in improving the performance of their countries' health systems. A desire for real progress and a recognition of important gaps in the information needed to undertake change led to political commitment and support across countries for a focused cross-national effort. The three-year initiative provided member countries with multiple opportunities to participate in and learn from component studies focused on pressing health policy issues. Countries also benefited from the information and exchanges that occurred, first at the kick-off conference in Ottawa, Canada in November 2001, and at no fewer than 20 subsequent meetings of officials and experts in venues ranging from Paris to The Hague to New York.

Performance improvement requires grappling with difficult questions. What can be done to ensure that spending on health is affordable today and sustainable tomorrow? What is needed to improve the quality and safety of health care, and to ensure that health systems are responsive to the needs of patients and other stakeholders? How should equitable and timely access to necessary care be supported? And perhaps the most challenging question of all: what can be done to increase value for money?

The Health Project offered a means for officials in member countries to learn from each others' experiences in tackling these questions, to draw upon the best expertise available across OECD member countries and within the OECD Secretariat, and to break new ground to support health-system performance improvement in the future. It encompassed nearly a dozen studies addressing key policy issues pertaining to human resources in health care, new and emerging health technologies, long-term care, private health insurance, health-care cost control, equity of access across income groups, waiting times for elective surgery, and other topics that are central to the policy concerns of OECD member countries. It was not possible to address every issue important to Health Ministries in the course of the project, but the issues that were chosen were ones considered to be of the most pressing importance.

The Health Project built on the foundation of the OECD's work in health statistics and health policy that has been carried out under the purview of various committees and working parties across the OECD. An important contributor to the success of the Health Project was its horizontal approach. Work in progress was discussed by experts and Delegate groups with a variety of important perspectives on health policy issues. The Project benefited from the guidance and support of an Ad Hoc Group on Health, made up of Delegates from member countries, and the specialised expertise of various OECD directorates was employed in tackling issues. The Directorate for Employment, Labour and Social Affairs, took the lead in coordinating the work conducted in horizontal co-operation with the Economics Department, the Directorate for Science, Technology and Industry, and the Directorate for Financial and Enterprise Affairs.

From my own political experience, I know how significant the results of this project will be for policy makers at the most senior levels of government. There are no governments within the OECD or beyond which will not derive important benefits from this work as they all struggle to meet varying challenges in the field of health care. It is apparent that there are few one-off solutions or quick fixes. But this project has demonstrated that benchmarking within and across countries, and sharing information can bring new ideas together and help policy makers meet those challenges.

Donald J. Johnston
Secretary-General of the OECD

Preface

T*owards High-Performing Health Systems*, the final report on the OECD Health Project, presents key findings from studies conducted as part of the Health Project and other recent work on health at the OECD. The report synthesizes the studies' findings using a framework that corresponds to the main health policy goals shared by OECD countries: health care that is accessible and of high quality, and health systems that are responsive, affordable, and good value for money. The report offers lessons on the effects of various policies intended to manage the adoption and diffusion of health-related technology, address shortages of nurses and other health-care workers, increase the productivity of hospitals and physicians, manage the demand for health services, reduce waiting times for elective surgery, and foster the availability of affordable private health insurance coverage. In addition, it sheds new light on problems policy makers face, such as judging the appropriate level of health spending, assessing the appropriate role for private financing in health and long-term care systems, and evaluating the implications for health-system performance of waiting times for elective surgery.

The report draws upon analysis of health data and policy carried out in a number of directorates across the OECD during the course of the three-year Health Project, referencing many of the publications and working papers that were produced. Elizabeth Docteur was the principal author of this report. Gaëlle Balestat and Gabrielle Hodgson provided statistical assistance, and Victoria Braithwaite and Marianne Scarborough provided secretarial support. Contributions and comments were received from across the OECD Secretariat. The report also benefited from input by participants at meetings of the Ad Hoc Group on Health, where drafts of this report were discussed.

Table of contents

List of figures

List of tables

Executive summary

OECD countries have good reason to feel proud of their accomplishments in improving health. A child born in an OECD country in 2000 can expect to live nine years longer, on average, than someone born in 1960. Infant mortality is five times lower today than it was then. In the past four decades, the level of premature death – as measured by years of life lost before age 70 – has been cut by half.

Economic expansion and rising educational attainment have laid the foundation for better population health, but improvements in health care also deserve some credit. The recent past has seen major breakthroughs in prevention and treatment for conditions like heart disease, cancer, stroke and premature birth, to name but a few. And with new drugs, devices and procedures, we can treat conditions better than before. For example, minimally invasive new surgical techniques result in quicker and less painful recovery for patients, and some who were not formerly candidates for surgery can now be treated.

In most countries, universal health-care coverage – whether public or privately financed – not only provides financial security against the costs of serious illness, but also promotes access to up-to-date treatments and preventive services. By 2001, more than two-thirds of OECD countries had achieved rates greater than 90% for childhood immunisation against measles, compared with only a third of countries ten years earlier. As a direct result of such improvements in health systems and health care, people are living longer and healthier lives.

Naturally, these gains do not come cheap. The most recent data show health-related spending to be more than 8% of GDP on average for the OECD area, and exceeding 10% in the United States, Switzerland and Germany. Compare this with 1970, when health care spending represented an average of just 5% of GDP in OECD countries. Much of this increase can be attributed to progress in medicine and the concurrent rise in expectations for health care. Simply put, advances in technology mean that we can do much more and so we expect more, but we must pay more, too.

Spending more is not necessarily a problem, particularly if the added benefits exceed the extra costs. But since three-quarters of OECD health spending comes from the public purse, government budgets are feeling the pinch. Even in the United States, where the private sector plays an unusually large role in financing, public expenditure on health represents 6% of GDP, comparable to what the average OECD country spends publicly on health.

The trouble is that upward pressures on health spending are unrelenting, reflecting continued advances in health care and increased demand from ageing populations. At the same time, the share of the population in its working years will decrease, straining public finances still further.

While richer countries tend to spend more on health, there is still great variation in spending among countries with comparable incomes. Even more importantly, the highest spending systems are not necessarily the ones that do best in meeting performance goals.

Cost and financing challenges aside, the public is increasingly aware that opportunities abound to improve the performance of health systems still further. Policy makers in OECD countries are faced with a large and growing demand to make health systems more responsive to the consumers and patients they serve, to improve the quality of care, and to address disparities in health and access to care. Is it possible to do better without raising cost pressure?

Health systems differ in their design, in the amounts and types of resources they use, and in the health outcomes and other results they attain. But health policy makers share common goals and can learn from each other's experiences as to what works – and what does not – when making changes to health systems intended to improve performance. The three-year OECD Health Project has sought to add to the evidence base and provide guidance that policy makers can adapt to their own national circumstances for use in their efforts to improve health-system performance.

High-quality health care and prevention

Big differences across countries in life expectancy and other indicators of health suggest that for many countries, if not all, further gains are possible. The extent of variation raises questions, together with expectations. For instance, why, in 1999, did Sweden and Japan have infant mortality rates of just 3.4 per 1 000 live births, while New Zealand and the United States reported rates over twice as high (7.2 and 7.7, respectively)? Why did 65 year-old women living in Ireland or Poland have an average life expectancy of less than 18 years in 2000, while women in Japan, Switzerland and France could expect to live three or more years longer than that?

Large differences in health status also exist between population groups within countries. These may be partly caused by barriers in access to needed services that affect disadvantaged populations disproportionately.

It is important not to overlook opportunities to promote better health through policy levers that fall outside the traditional purview of health policy makers. For instance, given the health impact of injuries and illnesses that are influenced by environmental and risk factors, improving health also means addressing factors such as violence, accident prevention and worker safety, road traffic enforcement, and the use of drugs, alcohol and tobacco.

Moreover, systems focused on curing illnesses today can miss opportunities to prevent illness and disability tomorrow. In fact, just 5 cents out of every health care dollar is spent on initiatives designed to keep people healthy. Yet population health has improved thanks to preventive measures like public awareness campaigns, regulation and taxation (in the case of tobacco, for example). Notable is the dramatic reduction in rates of smoking that has taken place in most OECD countries since the 1960s, leading to a decline in the incidence of lung cancer. But new threats have emerged, with the recent dramatic rise in obesity being a particular concern. Obesity raises the risk for chronic conditions ranging from diabetes to dementia, so the rapid growth in the share of obese adults foretells health problems in years to come. Stepped-up attention to prevention strategies is highly desirable in light of the difficulty in treating obesity.

One of the most important developments in health care over the past decade has been a popular awakening to problems of quality. In fact, across OECD countries, there is a large and expanding bank of evidence of very serious shortcomings in quality that result in unnecessary deaths, disability, and poor health, and that add to costs. The problems are of three types. First, some services are provided when, according to the standards of medical evidence, they should not be. Studies of elective surgeries like coronary artery bypass grafts show that a significant minority of certain procedures occur when the patient is not an appropriate candidate. This leads to an unnecessary exposure to health risks as well as wasted resources. A second type of quality problem is that patients who could benefit from certain basic services do not always get them. For example, medicines to control hypertension are often not prescribed when they should be, leading to inferior outcomes and higher costs later on. Aspirin is not prescribed to heart-attack patients often enough, even though it is a low-cost and effective way to reduce the risk of another heart attack. Yet a third type of quality problem arises from care delivered in a technically poor or erroneous manner. Examples here include wrong-site surgeries and mistakes in administering medicine.

Differences across countries in outcomes for conditions like stroke, heart attack and breast cancer might be explained by the intensity of treatments, the technical quality of care, the organisation and co-ordination of care, and influences outside the health system. More data on potential explanatory factors, such as prevention and screening, are needed to explore these possibilities.

Many OECD countries have started to monitor indicators of health-care quality, often for benchmarking purposes as part of broader efforts to track and improve health-system performance. In most countries, attention has first focused on the quality of hospital care, but initiatives to evaluate other health and long-term care settings are also under way. Such efforts can be strengthened by developing tools like clinical practice guidelines and performance standards that promote the practice of evidence-based medicine.

Better systems for recording and tracking data on patients, health and health care are essential for big leaps in quality improvement to be made. Paper medical records, prescriptions, and test reports do not support accuracy, access or sharing of information. Where they have been implemented, automated health information systems have had a positive impact on both health-care quality and cost. For example, hospitals in Australia and the United States that have adopted automated systems for placing medication orders in hospitals have achieved marked reductions in the rate of medication errors and related patient injuries, resulting in measurable improvements in quality and shorter lengths of stay.

Physicians and hospitals need to be given incentives to take on the cost of investing in automated data systems and the other steps needed to improve health-care quality. The economic and administrative incentives that are now in place sometimes actually discourage providers from doing the best thing. For example, in some countries, many unnecessary and inappropriate tests are prescribed because of the incentives set up by medical malpractice liability systems. Correcting such inappropriate incentives – and replacing them with ones that reward practice of evidence-based medicine – is essential to foster high-quality care.

Accessible health care

Concerns have been voiced in a number of OECD countries that a gap may be looming between demand for and supply of the services of physicians and nurses. Indeed, shortages have already appeared in a number of OECD countries. Despite increasing demand for services, supply is projected to fall, or at best to grow slowly (in the absence of countermeasures) as a result of societal trends to reduce work hours and retire early, physician workforce ageing, and diminished interest in nursing, relative to other professions.

Some countries are already seeking to increase the number and the productivity of physicians and nurses in their workforces. Strategies for training, retention, and recruitment from abroad have been used with varying degrees of success to increase the number of doctors. Increasing the nursing workforce has proved difficult, but there is room for more experimentation with approaches such as increasing nurse pay, improving working conditions and improving nurse education and training programmes.

Although ensuring comprehensive coverage of core services and minimising financial and other barriers to access have proven effective in promoting equitable use of health services, inequities in service use persist in some countries. These reflect factors such as the impact of user fees on lower-income groups, differences in insurance coverage across the population, and so on. The outcome can be poorer health, which further fuels economic isolation and social exclusion. Other types of inequities, such as disparities in the timeliness of service provision, can be the by-product of policies intended to foster a high degree of consumer choice.

Health policy changes alone may be insufficient to close gaps in health status for some disadvantaged groups, to the extent such disparities are symptoms of problems like poverty and social exclusion. However, experience shows that policy interventions can mitigate income-related inequities in access to care, where they exist, although this can be costly. In France, for example, the introduction of publicly financed coverage of cost-sharing for the poor has considerably reduced the pro-rich bias in the use of specialist services.

Medical advances offer chances to improve patient care and health outcomes, but they can increase aggregate costs as well. Uncertainty regarding costs and benefits, which is often the case, creates a dilemma for decision makers. Countries differ greatly in how decisions to adopt and pay for new heath-related technology are made, and these in turn affect diffusion. Some emerging technologies, such as gene therapies, pose ethical challenges that can make decision-making even more difficult. The conditional approval of promising technologies, pending further study; rigorous technology assessment practices; and use of transparent processes for decision-making, can all help in coping with uncertainty.

Responsive systems that satisfy health-care patients and consumers

Health systems can do more to meet the expectations and preferences of patients and consumers of health care. OECD work has identified policies that reduce waiting times for elective surgery and improve long-term care, two major sources of dissatisfaction in OECD countries. Also, offering choice in health coverage can result in a more responsive health system.

In at least a dozen countries, waiting times for elective surgery are viewed as excessive. Moderate waiting times do not appear to have negative effects on health outcomes, but they do affect quality of life; also, those waiting in discomfort remain less productive at work.

Countries wishing to reduce waiting times generally need to increase either the capacity or the productivity of their health-care systems. Costs will probably increase, though, since countries with long waiting times tend to have lower spending on health and fewer acute-care hospital beds. They also tend not to use fee-for-service payments for doctors and discharge-based payments for hospitals, which encourage productivity. And waiting times tend to be longest in those countries with fewer doctors per head. Nevertheless, if the supply of surgery is judged to be adequate, waiting times can also be reduced by ensuring that patients are not added to waiting lists unless (or until) their need exceeds a threshold level, while those with greatest need are assured of timely services.

A number of countries are experimenting with policies to provide consumers with more choice in long-term care services and to help patients get care at home, rather than in an institution, when feasible. Some countries provide funds to be spent upon such care, rather than payment for covered services, and such funds may be used to support family caregiving in most cases. This yields increased flexibility and control over services received, and reduced feelings of dependency. However, consumer-directed spending policies are likely to be more expensive than traditional approaches.

The availability of publicly or privately financed options for health coverage, in and of itself, can create more consumer choice. Furthermore, a health system in which multiple insurers are free to innovate can evolve in line with consumer preferences. But as with other benefits, choice has a cost. Compared with systems that feature just a single payer for health services or an integrated system of financing and delivery of care, multi-payer systems can raise spending pressure and make it difficult to maintain equity in access and financing.

Sustainable costs and financing

Systems that rely on contributions by working people for their financing will come under particular pressure as populations age and the share of the population participating in the workforce drops. Using general taxation revenues to finance expansion of health-care provision increases the burden on taxpayers or detracts from other publicly financed services and programmes. In order to relieve future public-financing pressure, individuals may be called upon to play a larger role in financing their own health care.

Cost-sharing requirements for users of health services can reduce the burden on public financing systems. But major savings from user fees are unlikely, particularly as vulnerable populations must be exempted to avoid restrictions on access that could be costly in the long run. Such exemptions impose administrative costs. Apart from this, consumers are likely to skimp on preventive care and appropriate treatments unless they are given incentives to do otherwise. Complementary private health insurance can help to ensure access to care where cost-sharing requirements are large. But it can drive up consumer demand and overall costs at the same time.

Private health insurance can offset some of the costs that would otherwise be borne publicly. However, subsidies are sometimes needed to encourage purchase of insurance and other interventions may be needed to promote the use of privately financed services by those with publicly financed coverage who are also privately insured. Even in countries where a sizeable share of the population is privately insured, private health insurance has tended to represent a relatively low share of total health spending, as it often concentrates on minor risks, rather than more costly cases and treatments.

Private health insurance premiums are a regressive source of financing compared with income-based taxes or social insurance contributions. When premiums reflect health-status factors, they may be as regressive as direct out-of-pocket payments, but they do nonetheless provide individuals with a means of pooling health-care risks and avoiding catastrophic expenditures. Government efforts to promote access to private health insurance through restrictions on risk selection or targeted subsidies can improve the equity of private health insurance markets, in terms of both financing and access to care, but at a cost.

Where private health insurance markets play a role in health financing, policy makers should carefully craft regulations and/or fiscal incentives to ensure that policy goals are met. Absent such interventions, private health insurance markets will fail to promote access to coverage for people with chronic conditions and other high-risk persons – as well as those with lower incomes. Additional interventions, such as standardisation of insurance products or other steps to help consumers understand the costs and benefits of insurance, can increase the potential of private insurance markets to make a positive contribution to health-system performance.

People need protection against the risk of incurring large expenses for long-term care, as for acute health-care and disability. Different approaches can work, such as mandatory public insurance (as in Luxembourg, Netherlands and Japan), a mix of public and mandatory private insurance (as in Germany), tax-funded care allowances (as in Austria) and tax-funded in-kind services (as in Sweden and Norway). The market for private long-term care insurance is small, but could increase with the right policy support.

Countries have slowed cost growth using a combination of budgetary and administrative controls over payments, prices and supply of services. Although sophisticated payment systems can be technically difficult to employ, there are numerous examples of successful systems – such as discharge-based payment systems for hospitals – that can promote productivity without harming outcomes. On the other hand, systems that keep health-sector wages and prices artificially low are likely to run into problems eventually, such as quality that has been bid down, difficulty with recruitment and retention of health-care practitioners, or shortfalls in the supply of services and innovative medical products.

Value for money in health systems

Ultimately, increasing efficiency may be the only way of reconciling rising demands for health care with public financing constraints. Cross-country data suggest that there is scope for improvement in the cost-effectiveness of health-care systems. This is because the health sector is typically characterised by market failures and heavy public intervention, both of which can generate excess or misallocated spending. The result is wasted resources and missed opportunities to improve health. In other words, changing how health funding is spent, rather than mere cost-cutting, is key to achieving better value.

Across the OECD, payment methods for hospitals, physicians, and other providers have moved away from cost-reimbursement, which encourages inefficiency, towards activity-based payments that reward productivity. But these systems also introduce risks, such as that of promoting service volume that is too high in some areas, and of low marginal benefit. They can under-value preventive services and treatments that reduce the need for expensive interventions later on. Far better would be payment methods that provide incentives to provide the right services at the right time, and that reward providers or organisations that contribute to realising performance goals, such as improved health outcomes. Some public and private payers are taking initial steps to improve payment incentives by offering bonus payments to health-care providers who meet certain quality standards, for example.

In systems where both financing and delivery of care is a public responsibility, efforts to distinguish the roles of health-care payers and providers, so as to allow markets to function and generate efficiencies from competition, have proved generally effective. In systems of any type, shifts in responsibility in health-care management or administration can also reduce waste and increase productivity. For instance, certain qualified nurse practitioners might undertake certain duties that are also performed by physicians, where safe and appropriate.

Nurses or general-practice physicians can serve as gatekeepers, assessing need for treatment and directing patients to the most appropriate care provider. With the Internet, patients can be informed about the costs, risks and expected outcomes for treatments. However, better information could either temper or increase demand. To promote value, patient cost-sharing requirements might be employed in a more discriminating manner, letting patients benefit financially from making cost-effective treatment choices.

In theory, systems featuring competing insurers (whether private or social) should promote a more efficient health system. In practice, it has proven difficult to establish value-based competition among insurers, as there is a tendency for competitors to try to attract healthier populations, who are less costly to insure. Policy measures such as banning discrimination in enrolment and implementing an experience-based system of risk compensation between insurers can counter this, but these same measures reduce incentives for insurers to manage costs.

Blunt cost-containment instruments can focus on short-term cost effects, failing to take into account possibilities to increase value over the longer-term through investment in new health-related technologies. Value-oriented management of technology can mean using technology assessment programmes and employing mechanisms like "value and cost agreements" between purchasers and manufacturers that take into account the effects of a new technology on patient outcomes and costs.

On track towards improved health-system performance

Health policy makers in OECD countries now know quite a bit about which tools and approaches can be used to accomplish many key policy objectives, such as controlling the rate of public spending growth, ensuring equitable access to care, improving health and preventing disease, and establishing equitable and sustainable financing for health and long-term care services. These tools and approaches have been used, with varying degrees of success, in reform efforts employed over the past several decades, providing a wealth of experience in both successes and failures from which to draw. In moving ahead, it is important to learn from past efforts to improve and to anticipate the many significant obstacles to successful change.

Health policy-making involves a careful balance of trade-offs, reflecting the weights assigned to a range of important goals and a great deal of uncertainty. The ultimate goal, certainly, is robust population health, but promoting health is not the only consideration. Health policy decisions can have considerable economic consequences, since the health sector is a strong and important component of the economies of OECD countries that provides extensive employment and profitable industry. Even when the tough choices are made, changing systems so as to improve performance is never easy, as the success of making change can be affected by the willingness of various stakeholders to embrace the proposed reforms. Given the speed of developments in medicine and evolution of health-care goals, reform of health systems is necessarily an ongoing, iterative process; there are few one-off solutions or quick fixes.

Recent work at the OECD has filled a number of knowledge gaps. But numerous important policy questions remain unanswered. Among the most urgent ones are: How can continued advances in medical technology be promoted and timely access be assured while managing public resources responsibly? How can innovation be guided in directions that best match health needs and priorities? What is the best way to ensure an adequate future supply of health workers? How can the economic motives of health-care providers be better aligned with goals for cost-effective health-care delivery? How can competitive market forces be better employed to increase the efficiency of health systems? Which approaches to medical professional liability can best deter negligence, compensate victims and encourage appropriate use of services?

Value for money is a moving target. Increasing value requires experimentation and conscientious performance measurement using actionable and specific indicators. Benchmarking within and across countries, and sharing information can help. Mutual observation is key to uncovering effective practices and the circumstance in which they work. Further work at the international level will, by bringing experience, evidence and new ideas together, help policy makers meet the challenges they face.

Introduction

OECD countries can be proud of the progress that has been made over the past three decades, a period of change and expansion for modern health systems. Most countries have attained universal coverage for a core set of health services and have taken great steps to ensure the accessibility of those services to the population. Population health status has improved steadily, even dramatically, driven largely by economic and social development, as well as concerted efforts to reduce the prevalence of risk factors and promote healthy living. Advances in medical capability and improvements in health care have had direct benefits in terms of both cure and prevention of disease.

Nevertheless, it is possible to improve the performance of health systems well beyond what has already been achieved. Serious and significant shortcomings in the quality of health care – at levels that would not be tolerated in other high-risk industries – have recently come to light. Patients and health-care consumers are demanding more from their health-care systems in terms of responsiveness to their expectations and preferences. In a number of countries, there are barriers that make it difficult for disadvantaged groups to realize equitable access to health-care services and the health improvements such access brings.

Furthermore, health systems are facing major cost and financing challenges. Health-care costs are growing faster than economies as a whole in many countries, posing problems for public budgets in particular, but also for some individuals in countries where a significant share of costs is borne privately. All signs indicate that countries must expect continued health cost-growth pressure, reflecting development of new treatments that affect supply, demand, and prices. Population ageing will have implications for the financing of health and long-term care services, and is likely to increase the demand for both, raising questions as to the affordability and sustainability of health systems. Health systems have great scope for improving efficiency by increasing productivity, reducing waste or enhancing the cost-effectiveness of care, yet achieving efficiency improvements has proven to be difficult.

This report presents work conducted by the OECD to assist policy makers in grappling with these challenges and seizing opportunities to improve performance. For each of five commonly held policy goals, it describes progress in improving performance, analyses current problems and identifies alternative approaches and best practices for addressing them. It begins by investigating the potential for further improvements in health through disease prevention and health-care quality improvement. It next considers approaches for resolving outstanding problems in fostering adequate access to care. The report then explores avenues for increasing the responsiveness of health systems. The cost and financing dilemma is examined in a following section. In the penultimate section, the prospects for increasing efficiency are considered. The report ends with a discussion of the key conclusions and advice for policy makers seeking to improve health-system performance.

ISBN 92-64-01555-8
Towards High-Performing Health Systems
© OECD 2004

Chapter 1

Better health through better care: the quest for quality

In every nation, people are living longer and healthier lives, thanks in part to the performance of their health systems. Access to health services is generally very good, facilitated by widespread availability of health services and comprehensive coverage of health-care costs in most countries. Nations are reaping the benefits from past public-health efforts, such as those to reduce smoking. And new medicines, procedures and technologies are continually being introduced to prevent and treat health conditions.

Yet chronic conditions – including ones, like obesity, that are related to behavioural and risk factors and ones, like dementia, that reflect population ageing – are on the rise, threatening population health. And there is growing evidence of very serious problems in the quality of health care – problems that result in unnecessary deaths, disability, and poor health, as well as wasted resources – and notable differences in the resulting outcomes, both across and within countries. Across the OECD, countries are recognising opportunities to further improve the health of their populations by improving the care furnished in their health systems.

Dramatic improvements in population health status

By most available measures, population health status has been improving steadily over time in OECD countries. For example, life expectancy at birth increased by an average of 8.6 years between 1960 and 2000 across all OECD countries (Figure 1.1). Infant mortality has declined dramatically, from an OECD average of 36.4 deaths per 1 000 live births in 1960 to 7.0 in 2000, an average annual decline of 4.6% since 1970 (Figure 1.2). In the last four decades, the level of premature death – as measured by years of life lost before age 70 – has been cut in half (OECD, 2003c).

Such improvements are due to rising standards of living and better education as well as advances in access to care and the capability of medicine.[1] Although improving health can be considered the major *raison d'être* of OECD health systems, measures of population health-status tend to be only indirect measures of health-system effectiveness. Life expectancy, infant mortality, and other such measures are highly influenced by social, environmental, and behavioural risk factors that are outside the direct control of healthcare providers and health policy makers.

The significant differences across countries in population health status that persist suggest that further advances are possible for many, if not all, OECD countries. One avenue for advancement is to assess the potential for changes in the context in which health systems operate. Many OECD countries could take significant steps to improve health by working outside of health-policy constructs, through changes to public policies that address issues such as violence, accident prevention and worker safety, driving regulations and traffic enforcement, and use of drugs, alcohol, and tobacco.

In addition, large differences in health status between population groups within countries have become a significant policy concern in countries where such problems are evident. For example, in the United States, there are marked differences in health status

Figure 1.1. **Gains in life expectancy at birth, total population, 1960-2000**

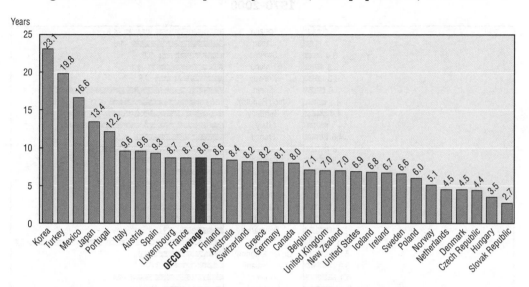

Note: Each country calculates its life expectancy according to methodologies that can vary somewhat. These differences in methodology can affect the comparability of reported life expectancy estimates, as different methods can change a country's life expectancy estimates by a fraction of a year. Life expectancy at birth for the total population is estimated by the OECD Secretariat for all countries, using the unweighted average of life expectancy of men and women.

Source: OECD Health Data 2003.

measures across racial and ethnic groups. Such differences have also been observed between indigenous and non-indigenous populations in Australia and Mexico. Health policy changes alone may be insufficient to close gaps in health status for some disadvantaged groups, to the extent such disparities are symptoms of problems like poverty and social exclusion. Rather, doing so requires a co-ordinated policy response to address root causes.

Disease prevention and health promotion initiatives

Some of the recent (as well as anticipated future) improvement in population health likely reflects major public-health improvement initiatives undertaken by OECD countries designed to prevent some of the most deadly and costly diseases. For example, more than two-thirds of OECD countries had achieved rates greater than 90% for childhood immunisation against measles by 2001, compared with only a third of countries ten years earlier, reflecting focused efforts to improve take-up rates in a number of countries (OECD, 2003c). Also, the proportion of daily smokers among the adult population has shown a marked decline over recent decades across most OECD countries, dropping on average from 36% in 1980 to 26% in 2000 (OECD, 2003d). Much of this decline can be attributed to policies aimed at reducing tobacco consumption through public awareness campaigns, advertising bans and increased taxation, in response to rising rates of tobacco-related diseases (World Bank, 1999). In addition, most OECD countries have developed national strategies for public health improvement that include immunisation, disease screening, and other steps to reduce population risk of developing diabetes, cancer and cardiovascular disease (Kalisch *et al.*, 1998). Nevertheless, interventions to promote health can be controversial and difficult to undertake. To the extent that ill-health arises from lifestyle choices, substance abuse and environmental and socio-economic circumstances, there are

Figure 1.2. **Infant mortality, 2000 and average annual declines in infant mortality, 1970-2000**

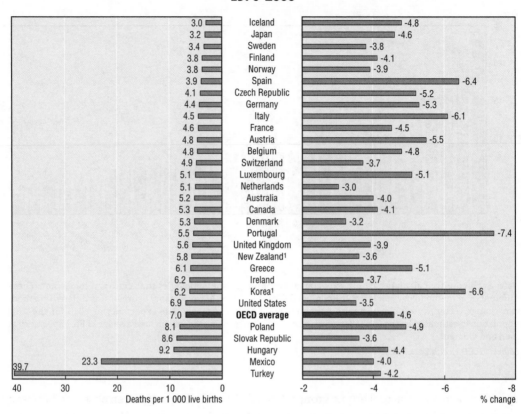

3.0	Iceland	-4.8
3.2	Japan	-4.6
3.4	Sweden	-3.8
3.8	Finland	-4.1
3.8	Norway	-3.9
3.9	Spain	-6.4
4.1	Czech Republic	-5.2
4.4	Germany	-5.3
4.5	Italy	-6.1
4.6	France	-4.5
4.8	Austria	-5.5
4.8	Belgium	-4.8
4.9	Switzerland	-3.7
5.1	Luxembourg	-5.1
5.1	Netherlands	-3.0
5.2	Australia	-4.0
5.3	Canada	-4.1
5.3	Denmark	-3.2
5.5	Portugal	-7.4
5.6	United Kingdom	-3.9
5.8	New Zealand[1]	-3.6
6.1	Greece	-5.1
6.2	Ireland	-3.7
6.2	Korea[1]	-6.6
6.9	United States	-3.5
7.0	**OECD average**	-4.6
8.1	Poland	-4.9
8.6	Slovak Republic	-3.6
9.2	Hungary	-4.4
23.3	Mexico	-4.0
39.7	Turkey	-4.2

Deaths per 1 000 live births — % change

Note: Some of the international variation in infant mortality rates is due to variations among countries in registering practices of premature infants (whether they are reported as live births or not). In several countries, such as the United States, Canada and the Nordic countries, very premature babies (with relatively low odds of survival) are registered as live births which increases mortality rates compared with other countries which do not register them as live births.
1. 1999.
Source: OECD Health Data 2003.

invariably complex issues and tradeoffs involved in public interventions that complicate policy making (Bennett, 2003).

Rising incidence of chronic health conditions

Across the OECD, general improvement in health status has been accompanied by a rise in the incidence of some chronic diseases, including asthma and diabetes, and expectations of significant increases in future prevalence. This can be attributed to several causes. One is high and rapidly rising levels of obesity, a risk factor for numerous chronic health conditions (see Box 1.1). Another is population ageing, given that older persons are more likely to have a chronic condition and more likely to have multiple such conditions. In addition, advances in medical technology are being used to treat acute illnesses and maintain a level of health and functioning that results in increased numbers of people living with chronic conditions (Partnership for Solutions, 2002). Finally, greater frequency and successful screening of diagnosing chronic conditions has resulted in earlier detection. As a result, more people are living with chronic conditions that used to grow to acute-care stages before diagnosis.

> ### Box 1.1. **Obesity: a public health threat**
>
> Obesity is a growing health concern in many countries. The rate of obesity has more than doubled over the past twenty years in Australia and the United States, while it has tripled in the United Kingdom (OECD, 2003d). More than 30% of the adult population in the United States is now considered to be obese. In Australia, Mexico and the United Kingdom, the rate has risen to more than 20%. In Continental European countries obesity rates are lower, but have also increased substantially over the past decade.
>
> Obesity is a known risk factor for diseases such as diabetes, hypertension, cardiovascular diseases, respiratory problems (such as asthma), musculoskeletal diseases (including arthritis), and even cognitive conditions, such as Alzheimer's disease. The economic and non-economic consequences of obesity are large. In the United States, a recent study estimated that obesity is associated with higher average health cost increases per year compared with the cost related to smoking (Sturm, 2002). In Canada, the total direct costs of obesity have been estimated to be over CAD 1.8 billion, or 2.4% of total health-care expenditure in 1997 (Birmingham *et al.*, 1999). And in the United Kingdom, obesity is estimated to result in 30 000 avoidable deaths per year (UK National Auditors Office, 2001).
>
> Policies to prevent or treat obesity aim to address its root causes, including bad nutrition and lack of physical activity. Governments in OECD countries are at various stages in experimenting with a range of policies and programmes to try to achieve the objectives of promoting better nutrition and physical activity. There is little doubt that the behavioural and environmental barriers to achieving the desired changes will be difficult to overcome.

Impact of ageing populations on health and disability status

Whether longer life expectancy is accompanied by good health and functional status for ageing populations has important implications for health-care systems. Fortunately, the evidence in at least a few OECD countries indicates that growth in life expectancy has not been accompanied by a growth in invalidity: severe disability rates in these countries appear to be falling as their populations age (Jacobzone *et al.*, 1998). Trends are not homogeneous across countries, however, and analysis by age/sex groups reveals some increases in disability rates over time. OECD countries are increasingly focusing their research and policy attention on conditions that affect the elderly disproportionately, including stroke, heart disease, and dementia.[2]

Variation in health outcomes across countries

Health outcomes, such as cancer survival rates and rates of disability among those with chronic conditions, reflect the effectiveness of care received more directly than do general measures of health status. In fact, high attainment in terms of population health status is not necessarily associated with best performance of health systems according to measures such as mortality amenable to health care (Nolte and McKee, 2003). As compared with population health status measures, measures of health outcomes are a relatively new focus of policy attention. Some research suggests that technological advances have been responsible for improvements in health outcomes for a number of health conditions (Cutler and McClellan, 2001). Although comparable data are limited at present, OECD studies making international comparisons of

Figure 1.3. **One-year case fatality rates for ischaemic stroke, 1998**

Percentage of patients who died within the first year following admission

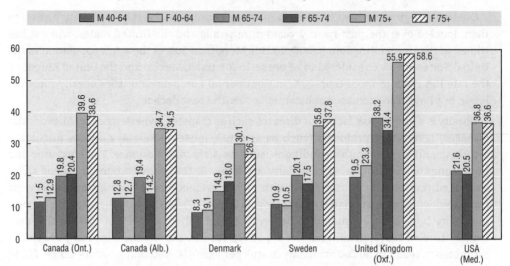

Note: Canadian data are from Alberta and Ontario, United Kingdom data are from the Oxford region, and United States data are from Medicare, which covers persons aged 65 years and older, as well as disabled persons under the age of 65.
Source: OECD (2003b).

Box 1.2. **Does waiting for elective surgery result in worse health outcomes?**

In general, people waiting for elective surgery are suffering from conditions which, despite not requiring urgent treatment, are progressive, such as stable coronary artery disease, arthritic hips and cataracts. Surgery candidates may be suffering from pain, disability, anxiety and even risk of death while they wait. Associated reductions in quality of life and any lost productivity due to inability to work must be taken into account when assessing the social and economic impact of waiting.

Studies of patients in those countries where waiting times are moderate (3 or 6 months, depending on the condition) have found little evidence to suggest that patients' health or surgical outcomes worsen as a result of waiting for elective surgery.[1] Longer waiting may be more problematic. For example, a study of patients on the waiting list for total hip replacement at one UK hospital found evidence of significant deterioration that increased with longer waiting. The median wait, here, was about one year (Kili *et al.*, 2003). Similarly, a UK study of patients waiting for varicose vein surgery found "considerable deterioration" in their condition while waiting for surgery (Sarin *et al.*, 1993). In this case, the median wait was 20 months. However, neither of these studies addressed the question of whether (long) waiting affected the final outcome of treatment.

Countries can minimise the health risks associated with "excessive" waiting by raising surgical capacity and productivity, and by supporting surgeons' efforts to monitor and reprioritise patients according to clinical need[2] (Hurst and Siciliani, 2003). For example, Denmark raised its capacity to provide revascularisation procedures steeply in the mid-1990s following the Danish "Heart Plan". Waiting times fell sharply. Mortality within 28 days after admission for a heart attack fell by about 30% in the following six years (although better drugs are likely to have played a part in this).

1. For example, see a Canadian study by Cox *et al.* (1996) and one from Sweden by Nilsdotter and Lohmander (2002).
2. A common policy is to impose maximum waiting times where there are queues for elective surgery, but that may interfere with surgeons' ability to prioritise patients on the basis of clinical need.

outcomes found significant differences in outcomes for conditions such as acute myocardial infarction (fatality rates and readmission rates), ischaemic stroke (fatality rates) (see Figure 1.3) and breast cancer (survival rates and mortality rates) (Moïse, 2003; Moon, 2003a; Hughes, 2003). Other studies of post-surgical mortality and cancer survival have also documented differences across countries (Roos et al., 1990; Roos et al., 1992; US General Accounting Office, 1994). Differences in outcomes may relate to differences across countries in the intensity of treatments for conditions, the technical quality of care furnished, the organisation and co-ordination of care, or influences outside the health system (see Box 1.2). Improved data – including more and better information on outcomes across the full continuum of care, as well as more data describing potential explanatory factors, such as preventive service use and screening – are essential to explore these possibilities (Moon, 2003b).

Significant shortcomings in health-care quality

A large and growing body of evidence points to the existence of substantial problems with the quality of medical care, indicating that services are overused, underused and delivered in a technically poor manner (Chassin and Galvin, 1998; Newhouse, 2002). Although uncertainty and lack of evidence in medicine play a role in observed variation in practice,[3] the degree of arbitrariness and inconsistency in medical decisions and their execution by far exceeds what could be expected because of these factors alone. Even where valid and well-known standards for practice exist, very often these standards are not met, as shown by examples below.

Inappropriate use of procedures

Research beginning in the 1980s has shown that a substantial part of surgical and interventional procedures, like coronary artery bypass grafting (CABG) or coronary angiography, is performed for indications for which the scientific evidence suggests that the risks outweigh the expected benefit. For example, an early study in this vein of research showed that 14% of all CABG procedures in three randomly chosen US hospitals could be labelled inappropriate (Winslow et al., 1988).[4] Comparable results have been found in other countries, even though their overall procedure rates tend to be much lower. In Sweden and the United Kingdom, researchers classified 10% and 16%, respectively, of CABG surgeries as inappropriate (Bernstein et al., 1999; Gray et al., 1990).

Under-use of accepted services

Universally accepted and widely known treatment standards are not routinely followed in daily medical practice. For example, there is uncontroversial evidence that patients benefit substantially from treatment with aspirin and beta-blockers after acute myocardial infarction. But only 84% and 72%, respectively, of patients are prescribed these drugs upon discharge from US hospitals (Jencks et al., 2000). A recent study found significant differences across five European countries (England, Italy, Germany, Spain and Sweden), the United States and Canada in the treatment and control of hypertension (Wolf-Maier et al., 2004). At the 140/90 mm Hg cutpoint, for example, two-thirds to three-quarters of the hypertensives in Canada and Europe were untreated, compared with slightly less than half in the United States. The researchers note that low treatment and control rates in Europe, combined with a higher prevalence of hypertension, could contribute to a higher burden of cardiovascular disease risk attributable to elevated blood pressure compared with that in North America.

Medical errors

The discovery of an alarmingly high rate of errors during the delivery of medical care has greatly increased the awareness of quality problems for policy makers, medical professionals and the public. Adverse events, like wrong-site surgery or medication errors, occur in 1-3% of all hospital admissions, according to studies from a variety of countries (Leape, 1994; Institute of Medicine, 1999; Schiøler et al., 2001). Estimates from the United States suggest that more people die from medical errors than from traffic injuries or breast cancer (Institute of Medicine, 1999). Such an error rate would be perceived as disastrous in other high-risk industries, like aviation. Here, even a failure rate of 0.1% is viewed as unacceptable, as it would translate, for example, into two unsafe plane landings each day at the Chicago O'Hare Airport (Deming, 1987 quoted in Leape, 1994).

Systemic causes of health-care quality problems

Health-care quality problems are believed to be primarily systemic in nature, with only a minority resulting from malfeasance or negligence on the part of individuals, organisations or institutions (Institute of Medicine, 2001). Medical science has advanced at an unprecedented rate during the past half-century. Health care has grown increasingly complex, with more to know, more to do, more to manage and monitor, and more people involved than ever before. Faced with such rapid changes, health-care delivery systems have fallen far short in their ability to translate knowledge into practice and to apply new technology safely and appropriately.

Today's health-care delivery systems are not organised in ways that promote best quality. Service delivery is largely uncoordinated, requiring steps and patient "hand-offs" that slow down care and decrease rather than improve safety. These transitions in care waste resources, lead to loss of information, and fail to build on the strengths of all health professionals involved to ensure that care is appropriate, timely, and safe. Organisational problems are particularly apparent regarding chronic conditions. The prevalence of patients afflicted with multiple chronic conditions strongly suggests the potential value of more sophisticated mechanisms to co-ordinate care. Yet health-care organisations, hospitals, and physicians typically operate as separate "silos", acting without the benefit of complete information about the patient's condition, medical history, services provided in other settings, or medications prescribed by other clinicians.

A number of factors combine to thwart change. Payments to health-care providers by and large reflect the volume of services delivered or the costs incurred in health-care provision, rather than appropriateness of care or health outcomes. The economic incentives of providers are not generally aligned with the goals of disease prevention and health maintenance. In a few countries in particular, defensive medicine, motivated by professional liability considerations, may encourage overuse of services such as diagnostic tests, irrespective of need, and may also provide incentives to cover up medical errors, rather than report them so that the experience can be used to avert similar future mistakes.

The health and economic impact of health-care quality problems

The health and economic toll of health-care quality problems is likely to be large, but partly hidden. Among the cost drivers are unnecessary diagnostic tests and procedures that add cost at little or no potential benefit. When the inappropriate care is an invasive procedure or surgery, patients are exposed unnecessarily to health risks in addition to the cost. Errors often result in patient injuries that extend hospital stays or require further treatment, adding to costs. For example, annual US hospital expenses to treat patients who suffer adverse drug events during hospitalization are estimated at between USD 1.56 and USD 5.6 billion annually (Agency for Healthcare Research and Quality, 2001). This estimate does not include the costs associated with additional hospital admissions, malpractice and litigation costs, or injuries to patients. Other costs incurred may also not be evident in health system accounts, including reduced productivity and days of work lost.

On the other hand, improving quality will undoubtedly have its own cost, at least in the short run. Increasing the rate at which patients get appropriate services when they need them will require additional resources or improved productivity. And making the system changes needed to improve quality requires up-front investments and resources to operate organisations and programs focused on improvement. Returns to investment over time are potentially large and should offset these up-front costs.

Tools and strategies for health-care quality improvement

The very fact that policy makers perceive a need to address the issue of quality of care represents a paradigm shift, as it was formerly taken for granted that the institutions of professional self-regulation would ensure adequate quality. However, both news-making incidents and research-based evidence of problems have raised questions as to whether this traditional societal arrangement is still viable in the face of the changing nature of medicine and changed ideas about accountability (see Box 1.3). As a consequence, many countries have begun to introduce new programmes, activities, and standards in the area of quality monitoring and improvement with the goal of making health care safer and more effective.

Major initiatives, such as the development of indicator frameworks to benchmark providers and the creation of new institutions to monitor and improve quality, have been launched in OECD countries (see Box 1.4). While these developments have often resulted in a greater role for the government as well as for purchasers and the public, the medical profession and its institutions are usually key participants.

Many OECD countries have instituted national strategies to begin to collect indicators of health-care quality, often for benchmarking purposes in a performance measurement setting. Those efforts have brought about much progress in implementing indicators of the quality of care furnished by specific types of providers, such as hospitals or physicians, and on the national level. In most countries, quality measurement and improvement initiatives have begun with a focus on the hospital sector, but approaches to monitor and improve care at the physician level and in the post-acute and long-term care settings are also under way (see Box 1.5). Such initiatives are strengthened by recent investments in tools that can be used to facilitate improvement in the quality of care delivered, such as information technology applications that will support physician decision making and provide large databases for quality-oriented research. Notably, there is much work under way to translate evidence from clinical research, health services research studies, and technology assessment findings into clinical practice guidelines and performance standards that can be used to promote practice of evidence-based medicine. Efforts have not been in existence for long enough to generalize as to their impact, but there is hope that the dynamic nature of this policy area will lead to innovative models and best practices in quality monitoring and improvement.

Box 1.3. **Improving health-care quality: policy options**

Scandals in several OECD countries have cast doubt on the institutions of professional self-regulation. Although the medical profession had formerly argued that these were caused by failures of individuals, rather than of professional institutions, there is growing evidence that the problems are systemic in nature and need to be addressed as such. This raises the question whether the best response can be found in reforms to the institutions of professional self-regulation, in the introduction of expert intermediaries (e.g. regulators, entities acting on behalf of purchasers) to safeguard quality, or in creating an environment in which competition among providers occurs partly on the basis of quality. The first option leaves responsibility for quality assurance with the medical profession, but would replace the former trust in the profession with trust in particular institutional arrangements that the profession puts in place. The second two options move away from the traditional division of responsibilities, the first by introducing intermediaries to act on behalf of patients or consumers and the second by empowering patients or consumers themselves to incorporate quality into their decisions on medical providers.

Obviously, these three options are not mutually exclusive but may be combined into an overall policy to improve quality of care and patient safety. The appropriate approach depends on the context and the historical structure of each health system. In particular, it needs to be consistent with societal values and attitudes, such as the relative weights placed on efficiency and equity, and the prevailing view on how responsibility is allocated to individuals or the state. Reforms will also raise difficult technical and political issues. For example, crafting a quality monitoring system requires substantial technical skills with respect to design of measures, adjustment for patient risk, and interpretation and presentation of information, as well as investment in research, data collection, information technology and human capital. Early experiments with consumer empowerment have uncovered an array of challenges in communicating technical information and making it salient to decision-making. Thus, the expected cost of, and returns on, those investments need to be taken into consideration. And even the most skilfully designed system is likely to encounter political resistance by stakeholders.

OECD countries offer examples of successful quality improvement from which some common themes emerge (Mattke, 2004). Regardless of whether the profession, a government agency or a private enterprise started the effort, successful efforts all share the features of an interdisciplinary approach, heavy reliance on data and measurement and strong leadership. Recent experiences are very encouraging, but applying such innovative models to the practice of medicine on a broader scale remains difficult and the challenge of achieving the necessary transformation should not be underestimated, as it will require fundamental changes in the organisation and culture of the medical profession.

Better data and information systems are needed to drive and support improvement

Paper medical records, prescriptions, and test reports rely on an outdated form of technology that does not support accuracy, access or sharing of information. Therefore, more investment in the areas of health data systems and electronic medical records is essential for quality improvement (Institute of Medicine, 1991). Barriers to progress include lack of universally agreed-upon standards for data collection and transmission and minimal financial incentives for physicians and other health-care providers to invest in electronic recordkeeping. Privacy considerations remain an important issue, and the digitisation of increasing amounts of genetic data raises some particularly difficult policy challenges.[5]

Box 1.4. **Quality oversight mechanisms: examples from OECD countries**

The US **National Committee for Quality Assurance** (NCQA) was founded as a self-regulatory body of the managed-care industry, but has become an independent and respected source of information on quality of care. Its best known product is the Health Plan Employer Data and Information Set (HEDIS), measures for assessing health-plan performance in quality of care, access to care and enrolee satisfaction. Under this system, in which about 90% of health plans participate, plans collect performance data and submit them to the NCQA, which then reports the measures back to the plan. Each plan may also authorize NCQA to release its data publicly, for use by employers and individual consumers in health-plan selection. Plans opting for public reporting perform better, on average (NCQA, 2003). NCQA also offers a voluntary accreditation system, in which about half of all plans participate, based partly on performance on the HEDIS measures and partly on an on-site review of clinical and administrative processes. More recently, in collaboration with medical specialty societies, NCQA has launched a recognition programme for individual physicians and group practices. To receive recognition, providers have to meet certain clinical performance criteria. So far, programmes exist for diabetes and for cardiovascular disease and stroke.

Two major initiatives are being prepared by the German **Federal Association of Statutory Health Insurance Physicians,** a self-regulatory body that has the legal mandate to ensure quality of care for sickness fund enrolees. The first is the development of a voluntary accreditation system for practices that focuses on quality of medical care. Each specialty will have specific criteria that will encompass structural information, processes and possibly outcomes. The second is the implementation of a real-time performance measurement system based on billing data. The system will consist of a set of process and outcomes indicators, which are constructed from the claims, along which each physician is continuously compared to a benchmark.

The **Commission for Health Improvement** (CHI) monitors the UK National Health Service (NHS), conducting reviews of NHS organisations to assess how well health care is managed. Its publicly available reports are meant to provide decision support for purchasers and regulators, as well as to show providers areas for improvement. In addition, CHI investigates incidents, conducts or commissions studies in health services research and fosters an exchange of best practices. In partnership with the Audit Commission, CHI is responsible for reviewing content and implementation progress of the National Service Frameworks, minimum standards of care for major diseases. CHI reports on areas of excellence and of shortcomings, but does not recommend or implement action plans. However, especially if substantial problems are detected, a follow-up survey will assess the response of management.

Nevertheless, there are examples of successful experience with digitised information systems in the health sector; for example, a US teaching hospital reported that it realised about USD 8.6 million in annual savings by switching to electronic medical records for its outpatient care (US General Accounting Office, 2003a). Other health-related applications of information and communications technology hold promise for improving effectiveness and cost-effectiveness of health-care delivery (see Box 1.6). For instance, hospitals in Australia and the United States that have adopted automated systems for placing medication orders in hospitals have achieved great reductions in the rate of medication errors as well as the patient injuries these entail, resulting in shorter lengths of stay and other measurable

Box 1.5. **The drive to improve quality of long-term care services**

The drive to raise standards in acute health care has been accompanied, in many countries, by governments taking a more active role in regulating and inspecting long-term care services. This has two aims: to reduce the risk of receiving poor-quality care, and to raise average standards of service.

Regulatory response to poor quality of institutional care

Quality regulations for institutional care have been made more comprehensive in several countries in recent years. From being minimum requirements for structure and process of care, covering safety of buildings, staffing ratios, etc., they have been developed into complex assessment and improvement instructions that include measures of outcomes, elements of continuous quality improvement (such as a commitment to continuous staff training), and new requirements for protecting patients' rights and privacy. There is also a trend away from a reliance on an initial inspection towards combining inspections with more demanding self-assessment and continuing care documentation by providers, with the aim of making quality assessment more reliable and quality improvement more transparent. These new regulations can impose significant resource requirements on providers in terms of capital investment, staff management and regulatory compliance.

Government initiatives to improve quality of long-term care include the re-accreditation process for care institutions in Australia following 1997 reforms, new and higher standards in Austria from 1994, the quality regulations put in place in Germany from 2002, and a new national regulator and national care standards in the UK in 2001. The process of accreditation of nursing homes under new regulations in a number of countries has revealed widespread shortcomings when measured against these standards. Failure rates of 40% or more for the initial assessment are not uncommon and few institutions seem able to report high ranking on all dimensions. A recent report on nursing homes in the United States noted improvement but found that one in five had serious deficiencies likely to place residents in danger or cause them immediate harm (US General Accounting Office, 2003b).

Deviations from quality standards are not uncommon in a number of countries. They include:

- inappropriate use of physical and pharmaceutical restraints;
- pressure ulcers (or bed sores);
- severe deficits in dementia care, such as inappropriate and/or insufficient support for eating and drinking; and
- a range of problems with lack of privacy and basic patient rights.

When such examples are uncovered and publicised, it pushes policy development in the direction of more detailed regulations covering more aspects of care. More experience is needed to be sure that this is the most effective way of dealing with a minority of low-quality providers. Most providers in most countries appear ready to act as partners in a process of steadily improving care, although this carries very obvious cost implications for users and for public budgets.

In a growing number of countries, the Internet now plays an important role in allowing consumer groups to gather information on unacceptable quality deficits and to increase the pressure on policy makers to implement strategies to prevent these. In a few cases, governments themselves use this channel of communication. For example, in Australia, summary reports of findings on individual providers are made available following each inspection. In the United States, the government puts information about the quality of nursing home care and home health care on the Internet for public use.

Box 1.5. The drive to improve quality of long-term care services *(cont.)*

New focus on quality of home health-care services

Regulation and monitoring of quality in the home-care market is a relatively new development. Policies for quality assessment and improvement in home care have recently been introduced in a number of countries (Australia, Canada, Germany, United Kingdom) and are being considered in others (Hungary, Japan). Surveys of both formal and informal home-care recipients have shown that satisfaction is relatively high compared with that of institutional care recipients and their families. On the other hand, quality problems in home care have been documented in surveys of health status and living conditions of dependent persons at home. The most frequent shortcomings are lack of consumer information about services available (Austria, United Kingdom) and limited access to services that support informal carers in their role as primary source of care. This was found even in countries with a generous public supply of formal home-care services. Evidence from these surveys indicates that access to a broad range of support services for informal carers, including respite care, training and counselling, is essential to maintaining quality of care at home and to prevent or mitigate adverse effects on the health of informal carers.

Source: OECD (2004b).

---

improvements in quality (Doolan and Bates, 2002). However, economic incentives are not aligned so as to ensure that hospitals and physicians benefit from these improvements and the expense of the systems can serve as a disincentive to invest in them.

Aligning incentives for quality improvement

Quality measurement and reporting systems may be used in a variety of ways to motivate performance improvements. Comparative information on the quality of care furnished by providers or health-care organisations is beginning to be incorporated in some accreditation programmes and regulatory oversight schemes, and is also being used in benchmarking as part of quality improvement programmes. In the United States and some other countries, such information is increasingly being made available to health-care purchasers, including consumers, for use in making value-based choices, thereby reducing information asymmetries that hamper markets for health services. However, to date there is limited evidence that purchasers (public or private insurers and patients) have incorporated such information into their purchasing decisions.

When private health insurance plays a primary role for a large majority of the population, release of plan-specific information on quality may provide incentives for insurers to compete based upon their contribution to the quality of the care they finance. During the 1990s, spurring such quality-based competition was an important underlying policy consideration in developing avenues for quality of care promotion in the United States. Efforts by voluntary accreditation organisations and large employers in the United States provide an example of such initiatives. A comprehensive review of the evidence on the impact of certain recent insurer-driven initiatives in the United States – such as performance-based and quality-based payments for providers – upon the quality of care delivery is needed. Certainly, many successful examples of improvements can be found. However, some evidence suggests that both employers and consumers failed to favour

Box 1.6. **Information and communications technology applications in health care**

Health systems are facing tremendous pressure to improve health quality, accessibility and outcomes, and to do so in a cost-effective manner. Health applications of information and communications technology (ICT) offer great potential to address these challenges. Examples include applications that stand to improve directly the care that is obtained by patients, such as electronic medical records that permit patients and doctors to have access to pertinent health and medical data, together with information pertaining to diagnosis and treatment, at the time care is provided. Other applications likely to be useful in this regard include consumer-oriented health web sites, electronic exchanges between patients and providers, patient monitoring and home care, remote consultation, medical imaging and clinical transactions. Other applications can accelerate health-related research and innovation via, for example, electronic biomedical databases, and improved opportunities for research collaboration. Furthermore, ICT can help with practitioner training and continuing medical education via distance learning.

There are significant impediments to effective ICT applications, mostly non-technical. Policy issues include the need for security, confidentiality and trust, modernisation of reimbursement rules to allow payment for electronically mediated services, and breaking down vertical barriers between different health delivery specialisations and health and administration services (OECD, 2004a). Nevertheless, many countries are making major investments in applying ICT more systematically to health. Recent examples include the UK multi-billion pound NHS electronic medical records initiative, and CAD 1.1 billion investment in the Canada Health Infoway.

As investment in information technologies in health expands rapidly, policy makers need a better understanding of the factors driving these developments and better information to guide and evaluate investment. However, a recent peer-reviewed study of more than 600 cost-related articles on telemedicine found that only 9% contained any cost-benefit data (Whitten et al., 2002). Globally, there is an urgent need for the development and application of consistent, rigorous, evidence-based methods to assess the value of ICTs in improving health outcomes.

health plans that showed better performance in health-care quality improvement, minimising insurers' incentives to invest in initiatives geared towards value-improvement.[6]

A few public and private purchasers in OECD countries have started to use financial incentives to encourage health-care providers (hospitals and physicians) to deliver high-quality services, or to reward desired health outcomes, a promising development in that such approaches usefully align economic incentives with desired outputs. For instance, programmes have been implemented in Australia and the United Kingdom that link financial rewards to the performance of general practitioners on a range of quality indicators. Systems of merit pay that reward physicians whose productivity exceeds expectations have been introduced in France, Germany, Sweden and the United Kingdom (Simoens and Hurst, 2004). The US Medicare programme launched in July 2003 a three-year pilot project that will provide higher reimbursement to hospitals that score well on 35 quality measures. Although there is clearly interest from many public and private payers in many countries, a number of technical obstacles and the potential to introduce undesired side-effects make design and implementation of such programmes very challenging.

Providers and others taking action to improve quality

Health-care providers and other stakeholders are responding to demand and incentives[7] to improve the quality of care in a great variety of ways. For instance, numerous quality improvement initiatives now flourish in the public and private sectors of many OECD countries. Some of these approaches rely on co-operation, sharing of data, and successful improvement experiences across providers, while others appear driven by value-based competition in which improvement tools or approaches may be considered proprietary information. Disease-management programmes, in which individuals with particular health conditions with high health or economic costs are given focused attention, co-ordination and guidance assistance by a nurse practitioner or other manager are increasingly used in some systems. Similarly, case-management approaches that target persons with multiple chronic or acute conditions that require great co-ordination across providers have been used. Efforts to integrate care on a vertical or horizontal basis have been driven, in part, by quality considerations. And initiatives to steer provision of high-risk services to hospitals that specialise in such (based on evidence linking volume and outcomes) have been undertaken side-by-side with broad-based quality-improvement programmes involving both high- and low-volume providers, reflecting the notion that maintaining local access is essential. The effectiveness of most of these approaches is not yet known, although highly successful examples of all of these approaches have been documented. So that policy makers can adopt approaches that suit the issues they face, both the effectiveness and the cost-effectiveness of these approaches need study.

Increasing information on cross-country differences in health-care quality

Datasets such as *OECD Health Data* that provide comparable information on health system characteristics and performance currently lack information on the technical quality of care furnished under those systems. This is a critical gap, as it limits the ability to undertake international benchmarking to inform design of evidence-based policies. Cross-country data on quality are essential to enhance international research on health-system performance and, in particular, to improve the ability to evaluate the cost-effectiveness of various institutional arrangements, resources and activities in the health sector.[8] Thus, at a time when national measurement systems are being implemented, there is an urgent need for international co-ordination. National activities do not lead to internationally comparable quality indicators, except by accident, as there is a lack of international agreement on the most promising indicators, and many alternative definitions, all scientifically sound, of each potential indicator could be adopted.

To fill this gap, the OECD instigated work to build on the efforts of several member countries and two smaller international collaborations to develop or identify indicators of health-care quality for use at the health-systems level. The first phase of the work is a developmental exercise that is testing the feasibility of collecting internationally comparable measures of the technical quality of care and of reporting those data to national and international policymakers and researchers. If successful, the long-term vision is to incorporate the quality indicators into *OECD Health Data* so as to enhance the scope of annually reported statistics and complement the currently available information on health-care systems in member countries.

Based on prior work and expert advice, the OECD adopted three criteria for selection of quality indicators: importance, scientific soundness, and feasibility. These criteria were used to select a set of quality indicators, drawing from those that had been selected by

Box 1.7. **Challenges and value of making cross-country comparisons of quality**

Comparing quality of care across countries is challenging because the methods by which data are collected, the extent to which the sample is representative of the underlying population, the definition of the population, the prevalence of disease, and the ways in which diseases are diagnosed and treated vary across countries. Valid and reliable data on intervention rates and health outcomes represent only the minimal level of information needed to make cross-country comparisons; in addition, information about data comparability, confounding variables and country-specific disease prevalence must be considered. Two examples below serve as illustrations.

Acute myocardial infarction mortality rates

In-hospital mortality for acute myocardial infarction (AMI) is an example of a quality indicator that has high policy relevance, a solid scientific background, wide data availability and the potential to be used as a tool for improving the quality of health care. AMI is a leading cause of death and one of the most frequent reasons for hospital admission in OECD countries. In recent years, AMI mortality has fallen dramatically, due in part to improvements in medical capability and care, including more rapid administration of thrombolytic agents, increased use of primary angioplasty, and more frequent administration of aspirin, beta blockers, and ACE inhibitors, and risk-factor reduction (Heidenreich and McClellan, 2001). Nevertheless, there is considerable evidence that clinical practice has fallen short of following clinical guidelines.[1]

In the first round of data reporting of OECD countries, 12 countries reported 30-day AMI mortality rates, ranging between 9% and 14%. Among higher-risk patients (those aged 75-89) this difference was larger (17% to 28%). Further work is required to resolve discordances in the age groups and years of the data reported. In addition, the question of the impact on comparability of limiting the measure to in-hospital deaths must be investigated further.

Asthma mortality rates

Asthma affected 5% of people and was responsible for about 3.4 deaths per 100 000 people in WHO Euro A countries in 2000. Deaths from asthma should be preventable if the condition is managed appropriately, making asthma mortality a potentially important quality indicator that is currently tracked by a number of OECD countries.

In the first round of data reporting, 16 OECD countries reported asthma mortality rates per 100 000 persons aged 5-39. The reported rates varied from less than 0.1 per 100 000 to 0.9 per 100 000. Differences in the coding of death certificates between countries could affect these mortality rates. A study of the accuracy of death-certificate coding for asthma found a low sensitivity (42%), but high specificity (99%), indicating that death certificates tend to underreport the true asthma mortality rate, although almost all deaths listed as caused by asthma are attributed correctly (Hunt *et al.*, 1993).

Despite comparability issues, however, international release of quality data still arguably can prove useful in drawing attention to areas for potential for improvement that could benefit from closer investigation. For example, New Zealand, which had a high asthma mortality rate relative to other countries, responded to earlier cross-country comparisons with a closer look at its asthma detection and treatment practices. Investigators discovered that the higher asthma mortality rate could be attributed in part to the use of high-dose fenoterol, a beta-agonist linked to asthma deaths (Beasley *et al.*, 1997). Following practice changes, New Zealand's asthma mortality rates have declined markedly in the past decade, approaching rates in other countries (Lanes *et al.*, 1997).

1. See, for example, EuroAspire I and II Group (2001), Bowker *et al.* (1996), and Jencks *et al.* (2003).

previous international collaborations. In response to perceived gaps in the comprehensiveness of the initial list, the OECD also convened panels of experts who recommended promising indicators in five clinical areas for further evaluation and possible future data collection.

Preliminary data were collected from 21 participating countries for the original indicators. The outcome of the initial data collection was encouraging in that, for every indicator, at least some of the responding countries could provide data. Not unexpectedly, availability was better for those indicators, such as cancer survival rates, for which data are commonly collected by national registries. But even for demanding measures, like "Diabetic Patients with Elevated HbA1c levels", which requires conducting blood tests in a population-based sample, data sources could be identified in three countries. Work is under way to assess comparability of the preliminary results and to identify avenues for improving comparability (see Box 1.7).

Approaches for improving health and health-care quality: summary of findings

Although health improvement is a fundamental goal of health systems, the most important determinants of population health status lie outside the immediate purview of health-care providers and health policy makers. In particular, the socio-economic and social context in which health systems operate deserves examination, as changes in behavioural or social factors might do more to improve health than could ever result from changes to health care or the health system made in isolation.

Attention to the quality of care is a relatively new policy concern, and the net effects of activity in this area on mortality, morbidity and quality of life are not yet known. Nevertheless, innovation in this area appears promising, and many changes, such as those designed to reduce medical injuries and decrease the provision of unnecessary care, stand to improve the cost-effectiveness of health-care delivery. Many countries have taken steps toward quality improvement, but more is needed in some countries, particularly in the area of long-term care.

The fact that such innovation relies upon development of systems for performance measurement and monitoring, including better systems for management of health data, is a positive development, in that these systems are likely to contribute to improvement in performance along an array of policy goals. Health applications of information and communication technology may facilitate needed progress in improving the systemic processes and organisation of health-care delivery. A key outstanding challenge for many health systems is to ensure that the economic and administrative incentives faced by providers and patients are aligned with policy objectives for improvement.

Notes

1. Other factors, such as better nutrition, sanitation and housing also play a role, particularly in countries with developing economies.

2. See A Disease-based Comparison of Health Systems (OECD, 2003b) for information on how OECD countries are coping with stroke, heart disease, and breast cancer. A forthcoming working paper (Moïse et al., 2004) considers health and long-term care issues for patients with dementia and Alzheimer's disease.

3. Evidence on appropriate clinical indications for undertaking procedures such as caesarean sections, tonsillectomy, and other common procedures is lacking, contributing to widespread variation in practice.

4. More recent US studies also document overuse of certain procedures. For example, a study drawing on data from the late 1990s found that 10.6% of carotid endarterectomy procedures performed in six US hospitals were inappropriate (Halm *et al.*, 2003).

5. The OECD held a workshop in Tokyo in February 2004 on issues of privacy and security with respect to human genetic research databases.

6. In the United States, efforts to provide consumers with information on quality and other dimensions of health-plan performance have had limited impact on consumer decision-making to date, partly because consumers do not find such information salient, questioning the insurer's role in ensuring quality, and find quality information technical and difficult to understand (Reilly *et al.*, 2002).

7. For example, high-profile media coverage of adverse events and malpractice litigation raised public demand for reform of hospital accreditation standards in Japan (Hirose *et al.*, 2003).

8. Absent data on the quality of health care, cross-country comparisons of relative efficiency are limited to productivity considerations, but no judgments as to whether productivity is optimised are possible. Quality information is necessary to assess the cost-effectiveness of health-care delivery.

ISBN 92-64-01555-8
Towards High-Performing Health Systems
© OECD 2004

Chapter 2

Access to care:
the quest to improve and maintain

A goal at the heart of health policy-making in OECD countries is achievement of adequate access to essential health-care services by all people on the basis of need. Many OECD countries endorse equity of service use as a metric of that adequacy, adopting a standard articulated as "equal care for equal need". Other countries accept variation in access to certain services, particularly those perceived as luxuries or not strictly medically necessary.

OECD countries have made tremendous progress in increasing access to health services over the past several decades. Such progress was driven first by initiatives to extend coverage for health-care costs across the full population and has continued with efforts to ensure timely, local availability of affordable services and to eliminate barriers to access. Nevertheless, disparities across population groups persist in many countries, a concern because of the implications for health and economic status of these groups. For those countries where access to services is considered adequate and equitable, maintaining this status tends to be an important policy consideration.

The situation with long-term care services is somewhat different. Informal care provided at home is still the most important source of long-term care. Localised problems in access to institutional care exist in some countries due to a shortage of long-term care providers, leading to long waits before entry to a nursing home, or the use of more costly hospital care as a fall-back. Reflecting patient preferences and other policy considerations, many countries are seeking to address this problem by further increasing the capacity to furnish care in the community setting, rather than expanding the supply of institutional care. To ensure that those who have a need for intensive care in an institution can obtain it, some countries have enhanced coverage of such needs while restricting subsidies for those with mild disabilities.

Given the importance of new medical technologies for preventing and treating health conditions, policy makers want to ensure appropriate access to new drugs, devices, and treatments. The important cost considerations associated with technological change make prudent decision-making critical. Prudent decision-making should take into account the effectiveness and efficiency of available options, as well as other considerations. This can be particularly challenging where necessary information is lacking. In the case of new and emerging health technologies, particularly the sophisticated and complex technologies that are in the pipeline today, the challenge will be even greater as ethical dimensions come to the forefront and both costs and benefits become increasingly hard to quantify.

Public coverage or private insurance is important to promote access to care and financial protection

In most countries, universal health-care coverage provides financial security against the costs of serious illness and promotes access to treatments and preventive services.

Most individuals have public coverage or private insurance for health care

Most OECD countries have long achieved close to universal coverage of their population for at least a core set of health services (Table 2.1). All but five OECD countries have publicly financed systems that provide universal or near-universal coverage[1]

Table 2.1. **Coverage by public schemes and private health insurance in OECD countries, 2000**

	Public health expenditure as % of THE[1]	Public system coverage[1]	Eligibility for public coverage[2]	PHI as % of THE[1]	Population covered by PHI, %[3]	Types of private coverage
Australia	68.9	100	All permanent residents are eligible for Medicare (the tax-financed public health insurance system). Eligible persons must enrol with Medicare before benefits can be paid.	7.3	44.9 40.3[4]	Duplicate, Complementary Supplementary
Austria	69.4	99	Almost all labour force participants and retirees are covered by a compulsory statutory health insurance. Social assistance claimants and prisoners receive health benefits and services from the state authorities. 1% are without coverage.	7.2	0.1 31.8	Primary (Substitute) Complementary, Supplementary
Belgium	72.1	99	Compulsory statutory health insurance includes one scheme for salaried workers and one scheme for the self-employed people (about 12% of the population in 1999). The latter excludes coverage of "minor risks" such as outpatient care, most physiotherapy, dental care and minor operations.	n.a.	57.5[a]	Primary (Principal), Complementary, Supplementary
Canada	70.9	100	All population is eligible for public coverage financed by Federal and Provincial taxation.	11.4	65.0 (est.)	Supplementary
Czech Republic	91.4	100	All permanent residents are eligible for statutory health insurance coverage.	0 (est.)	Negligible	Supplementary
Denmark	82.5	100	All population is eligible for public coverage financed by State, County and Municipal taxation.	1.6	28 (1998)	Complementary, Supplementary
Finland	75.1	100	All population is eligible for public coverage financed by State and Municipal taxation.	2.6	10	Duplicate, Complementary, Supplementary
France	75.8	99.9	The social security system provides coverage to all legal residents. 1% of the population is covered through the Couverture Maladie Universelle (CMU).	12.7	86.0 (92 including CMU)	Complementary, Supplementary
Germany	75	90.9	All employed people and their dependents are covered by statutory health insurance coverage. This does not include self-employed individuals and civil servants. Employees with an income above an income threshold can opt out of the social sickness fund system. Fulfilling certain requirements, social security insurees can choose to "stay in" the public system on a voluntary basis even if they are allowed to opt out of the system. Self-employed may also join on a voluntary basis.	12.6	18.2 of which: 9.1 9.1[b]	Primary (Substitute) Supplementary, Complementary
Greece	56.1	100	All population is eligible for public coverage, financed by a combination of taxation and social health insurance contributions.	n.a.	10[5]	Duplicate, Supplementary
Hungary	75.5	100	All permanent residents are eligible for statutory health insurance coverage. Only 1% of the population was not covered in 1999.	0.2	Negligible	Supplementary
Iceland	83.7	100	All permanent residents are eligible for statutory health insurance coverage.	0 (est.)	Negligible	Supplementary
Ireland	73.3	100	All resident population is eligible for public hospital coverage, financed by general taxation. Only about one third of the population with medical cards is eligible to GP and other outpatient coverage.	7.6	43.8	Duplicate, Complementary, Supplementary
Italy	73.4	100 (1997)	All population is covered by the National Health Service system, financed by general taxation.	0.9	15.6 (1999)[5]	Duplicate, Complementary, Supplementary
Japan	78.3	100	All population is covered by a statutory social health insurance system.	0.3	Negligible	n.a.
Korea	44.4	100	All population is covered by a statutory social health insurance system.	n.a.	n.a.	Supplementary
Luxembourg	87.8	99	All population is covered by a statutory social health insurance system, apart from civil servants and employees of international institutions (1%).	1.6	2.4	Complementary, Supplementary

Table 2.1. **Coverage by public schemes and private health insurance in OECD countries, 2000** (cont.)

	Public health expenditure as % of THE[1]	Public system coverage[1]	Eligibility for public coverage[2]	PHI as % of THE[1]	Population covered by PHI, %[3]	Types of private coverage
Mexico	47.9	45-55 (est.)[c]	Public social security schemes cover all the population working in the private formal sector and government workers, i.e. excluding independent self-employed workers, informal sector workers and unemployed people. From 2004, the System of Social Protection in Health offers a new public health insurance scheme that has been implemented to provide voluntary public health insurance to the population previously excluded from social security.	2.5 (2001)	2.8	Duplicate, Supplementary
Netherlands	63.4	75.6	Eligibility to statutory health insurance is determined by income. Individuals above a threshold are not covered (28.9% in 2000).	15.2	92 *of which:* 28.0 64 (est.)[b]	Primary (Principal) Supplementary
New Zealand	78	100	All population is eligible to public coverage financed by general taxation.	6.3	35[6]	Duplicate, Complementary, Supplementary
Norway	85.2	100	All population is eligible to public coverage financed by State, County and Municipal taxation.	0 (est.)	Negligible	n.a.
Poland	70	n.a.	All eligible groups are entitled to statutory health insurance cover. People who are not specified in the eligible groups by the Act of 6 February 1997 can purchase the social health insurance voluntarily.	n.a.	Negligible	Supplementary
Portugal	68.5	100	All population is covered by the National Health Service system, financed by general taxation.	1.5 (1997)	14.8	Duplicate, Complementary, Supplementary
Slovak Republic	89.4	100 (1999)	All population is covered by a statutory social health insurance system.	0 (est.)	Negligible	Supplementary
Spain	71.7	99.8 (1997)	Almost all the population is covered by the National Health System, financed by general taxation. Civil servants and their dependents are covered through a special scheme. A minor group of self-employed liberal professionals and employers are uncovered.	3.9	13 *of which:* 2.7 10.3[7]	Primary (Substitute, Principal) Duplicate, Supplementary
Sweden	85	100	All population is covered by a statutory social health insurance system, financed by local taxes and state grants.	n.a.	Negligible	Complementary, Supplementary
Switzerland	55.6	100[d]	All permanent residents are mandated to purchase basic health insurance.	10.5	80[d]	Supplementary
Turkey	71.9 (1998)	66 (1997)	Population coverage through three social security schemes for private sector employees, blue collar public sector employees, self-employed persons and retired civil servants.	0.7 (1994)	<2[8]	Complementary, Supplementary
United Kingdom	80.9	100	All UK residents are covered by the National Health Service system, financed by general taxation.	3.3 (1996)	10.0	Duplicate, Supplementary
United States	44.2	24.7	Individuals eligible to public programmes include those older than 64 and severely disabled (Medicare), poor or near poor (Medicaid) and poor children (SCHIP). Eligibility thresholds to Medicaid are set by states.	35.1	71.9	Primary (Principal) Supplementary, Complementary

Note: (est.): figures are estimated; CMU: "Couverture Maladie Universelle", a publicly financed programme providing complementary health insurance to eligible low-income groups. PHI: Private Health Insurance; THE: Total Health Expenditure; negligible indicates a proportion covered of less than 1%; n.a. indicates not available.

a) For Belgium, data include voluntary PHI policies for hospital care that are compulsorily offered by several sickness funds to their members, as well as PHI policies offered by commercial companies. They exclude policies for hospital care offered by sickness funds to their members, that guarantee insurees a limited lump sum (mostly less than 12.4 euros per day (Office de Contrôle des Mutualités et des Unions Nationales de Mutualités, 2002, *Rapport Annuel*, p. 81) and covered about 67% of the population in 2000.

b) For the Netherlands and Germany, the data refer to supplementary PHI policies purchased by individuals who belong to the social health insurance system. Some of the individuals with primary PHI are also covered by supplementary PHI policies, which are sometimes packaged with primary PHI policies.

Table 2.1. **Coverage by public schemes and private health insurance in OECD countries, 2000** (cont.)

c) These coverage figures relate to social security schemes, which include workers in the private formal sector and civil servants. Important to note that public health expenditure as a percentage of THE includes all public health spending, i.e. both social security spending and other public spending, such as resources used to finance health care provision for the uninsured population through the states' health services. Estimates vary depending on the source used; population survey data report lower figures, official administrative data report higher figures but no roster of individuals covered by the social security system is available.

d) For Switzerland, data on PHI refer only to voluntary private health insurance coverage. Mandatory health insurance covering the entire population is reported in *OECD Health Data* as public coverage, although it is a border line case.

Source: Specific data sources have been indicated below; information was also supplied by OECD member countries or obtained from official publications.

1. OECD *Health Data* 2003, 2nd edition, 2000 data unless otherwise indicated.
2. OECD PHI Regulatory Questionnaire, 2003 and other official sources.
3. OECD PHI Statistical Questionnaire, 2000 data, unless otherwise specified.
4. PHIAC (2002), *Operations of the Registered Health Benefits Organisations Annual Report 2001-02*. Data refer to June 2001.
5. Mossialos and Thomson (2002), *Voluntary Health Insurance in the European Union*.
6. European Observatory on Health Care Systems (2001), *Health Care Systems in Transition. New Zealand*.
7. Ministry of Health, Spain (2003), *National Health Survey 2001*. According to another estimate population coverage was 16.2% in 2002 (11.3% duplicate and 4.9% substitute) (Data from UNESPA, December 2003).
8. UK Trade and Investment, "Health Care and Medical Market in Turkey", *www.tradepartners.gov.uk/healthcare/turkey/profile/overview.shtml*; note that this figure does not distinguish between PHI alone and PHI offered as riders to life insurance policies.

Box 2.1. **Increasing access to health care: recent initiatives in OECD countries**

Some OECD countries have taken recent steps to increase access to care for disadvantaged groups through enhancing their coverage under publicly financed schemes. One notable example is the introduction in **France** in 2000 of the universal health coverage law, known as the *Couverture Maladie Universelle* (CMU). The CMU is a means-tested programme designed to promote access to care for low-income persons who do not have other complementary coverage. The CMU covers all co-payments for doctor consultations, hospital per diems, and glasses and dental prostheses, meaning that care is essentially free for CMU beneficiaries. About 8% of the French population was entitled to CMU benefits in 2002. The first assessments of the impact of the CMU on health-care utilisation indicate that the volume of services used by CMU beneficiaries increased, compared both to their pre-CMU level of consumption and to individuals whose income is too high to be entitled to CMU, but who do not have any complementary insurance. The rise in consumption was especially strong for specialist consultations, dental care and eye care. The health spending of CMU beneficiaries was estimated to be about 20% higher compared with people with no complementary insurance (DREES, 2003). The overall cost of the CMU was 1 200 million euros in 2002 (Fonds de Financement de la CMU, 2003).

In **Mexico**, only about half of the population had health insurance in 2000; the remainder of the population relied mainly on publicly provided services of uneven quality and availability, especially in rural areas. As part of the *National Health Program 2001-2006*, the government proposed a reform of the General Health Law to provide publicly financed health coverage to the almost 45 million people in Mexico who do not have coverage. The *National Health Program* also aims to address the issue of poor-quality services and long waiting times in the public sector.

In the **United States**, where private health insurance is the dominant form of coverage, more than one in seven people is uninsured. The options for increasing coverage are to expand existing public programmes or to facilitate additional purchase of private insurance. Initiatives of both types have been taken recently, representing efforts to target different segments of the uninsured population. For instance, the *State Children's Health Insurance Program* was created in 1997 to expand coverage for uninsured children ineligible for the existing Medicaid programme for the poor, and has reduced the share of children who are uninsured. The *Trade Act* of August 2002 provides a tax credit to subsidise private health insurance purchase by individuals who have been displaced by trade and retirees aged 55-64 who have lost retirement benefit due to employer bankruptcy. The current administration has also proposed broader tax credits for this purpose.

spanning at least doctor consultations and inpatient care. In two of the remaining countries (Germany and the Netherlands), private health insurance[2] serves as primary coverage for a share of the population, bringing the level of coverage up to near-universal levels, leaving three countries – Mexico, Turkey and the United States – with significant uninsured groups. In light of the role coverage plays in promoting access and financial protection, expansion of coverage has been put forward as a policy priority in all three countries and other countries have taken steps to improve the coverage provided to vulnerable populations (see Box 2.1).

Private health insurance plays different roles in OECD countries, ranging from primary to duplicate, complementary and supplementary coverage (Table 2.1). It represents the sole form of health coverage for significant population segments in Germany, the Netherlands, and the United States. In Australia, Ireland, Spain, and the United Kingdom, among others, private health insurance provides a private alternative to public coverage, furnishing privately insured persons with access to privately financed providers that may or may not be separate from public delivery systems. In France, the main function of private health insurance is to complement and top-up partial reimbursement by the social security system.[3] Most OECD countries also have private health insurance policies available to cover services that are not covered by public programmes.

A few countries have seen a notable rise in populations purchasing private health insurance in recent years.[4] In some cases, this has been triggered by economic growth and employer participation (*e.g.* Ireland); in others it may be attributed to government interventions (*e.g.* Australia). In several OECD countries, employers are taking on an increasing role in the offering of private health insurance and this may augment market size and the contribution of private health insurance to total financing. Markets with significant employer-sponsored insurance may experience better risk pooling.[5]

The prospect of introducing or expanding private health insurance coverage may raise concerns about whether affordable coverage will be available to all population groups, a particular issue where private health insurance plays a primary financing role for certain population groups (see Box 2.2). Policy interventions, such as regulation and subsidisation of private health insurance, can be used to address such problems.

Comprehensiveness of coverage varies

The range of health-care benefits furnished by publicly financed schemes varies across countries (Table 2.2). All cover doctor consultations and inpatient care. Most, with exceptions such as Canada[6] and the US Medicare programme,[7] cover prescription drugs. Fewer include dental care. The extent of cost sharing for services covered by public schemes also varies across countries. It ranges from zero or very low levels of cost sharing for doctor consultations and hospitalisation in many countries up to about 50% in Korea. In most countries, cost-sharing is higher for prescription drugs. In part reflecting such variation, the share of total household consumption represented by out-of-pocket spending on health care ranges widely across OECD countries, from 1% or less in the Czech Republic and the United Kingdom, to more than 4% in Korea, Mexico and Switzerland. However, the implications for access depend largely on how out-of-pocket costs are distributed across the population.

Coverage for long-term care services

There are considerable differences across countries in the means used to meet the cost of long-term care (Table 2.3). In many countries, long-term care has been defined as a part of the social-care sector rather than the health-care system. There is also a distinction between those providing access to long-term care based on need and at low cost to the user, in a similar way to health care (as in Norway and Sweden) and those in which long-term care is similar to social assistance, in that it is provided at public cost only where the user cannot pay for themselves (as in New Zealand, Spain, the United Kingdom and the United States). Some countries that traditionally have provided long-term care as a safety-net service to those unable to pay for their own care have modified the tests of income and assets to make the financial call on private assets more affordable (*e.g.* New Zealand, United Kingdom).

Box 2.2. **Policies to foster availability and affordability of private health insurance**

OECD countries with private health insurance (PHI) markets face challenges arising from certain characteristics of competitive, voluntary markets, including segregation by risk[1] and information asymmetries between insurance purchasers and sellers. Therefore, absent government interventions, some PHI markets offer limited or no policies for high-risk populations and coverage may not be affordable for some lower- and middle-income groups. These considerations apply broadly, but are of particular importance when PHI is the sole source of coverage for certain population groups, as in the United States, or when it is considered an important pillar of the health system, with significant levels of population coverage, as in the Netherlands.

In light of these concerns, governments in some countries have intervened to promote access to insurance. Financial incentives for the purchase of PHI may promote product affordability, but are often less targeted to address affordability for sicker populations. The impact of such incentives on levels of PHI purchase has varied. For example, there is debate in Australia around the extent to which a PHI premium rebate contributed to increased coverage, as opposed to other government policies. Furthermore, subsidies need to be significant in their amount to affect take-up. At the same time, the presence or absence of financial incentives has shaped PHI markets. Tax breaks have encouraged the employer market in the United States and, conversely, the fringe benefit tax has hindered development of the employer market in Australia.

Among the regulatory practices used to promote access to insurance is to require insurers to offer at least one product to high-risk persons and to accompany this requirement with restrictions on premiums, as is done in Germany and the Netherlands. While this does not promote risk pooling across insurer offerings, it does ensure access as well as participation by all insurers in promoting this access. Other practices include prohibitions on selective acceptance of enrolees by risk for all products, or separate coverage pools for those of high risk. Cross-subsidisation or risk equalisation mechanisms within or across insurers or insured populations may help assure the fair and equitable application of these standards across insurers or insured populations.

Independent bodies to adjudicate consumer concerns, combined with complaint response mechanisms operated or overseen by government, can help assure that consumer concerns are addressed and provide policy makers with feedback concerning possible areas for policy intervention. Such mechanisms exist in Ireland, Australia and many US states, where they provide assistance to consumers without requiring expensive legal action. They also help build confidence in the private insurance system.

The decision to impose standards to foster access to PHI markets – and the tools selected – depends upon the role of PHI in the health system and policy maker and cultural priorities – notably the level of tolerance for risk- and income-based differentials in access to PHI. Regulation carries a price, as it may limit the scope for insurers to innovate and respond to individual preferences in the development of their products and may restrict access to insurance if the regulation raises premiums above the value of such coverage to the healthier population (OECD, 2004c).

1. Risk-selection activities include insurers' restricted acceptance of applicants or exclusions on the coverage of high-risk persons that can result in reduced coverage of persons with significant health-care needs. Insurers or insurance products experience adverse selection when purchasers only buy coverage when they anticipate a need, or when they attract a disproportionate share of high-risk individuals. Both risk selection and adverse selection minimise the risk-sharing effect of insurance and may result in problems with available or affordable insurance for some people.

Table 2.2. **Cost-sharing policies in public schemes for basic health coverage[1]**

Degree of cost-sharing in per cent and in USD or EUR

	General practitioner	Specialist	Drugs	Inpatient care	X-ray and pathology
Australia	For 25% of bills, average of USD 5. General patient reimbursed 85% of schedule fee if not bulk billed.	For 71% of bills, average of USD 8. Patient reimbursed 85% of schedule fee if referred.	Maximum AUD 23.70 (around USD 18) per prescription for general patients for drugs on the PBS Scheme.	None.	Included in specialists' bills.
Austria	20% of the population pays between 10% and 20% of doctor's fee.	Same as for GPs.	USD 4.50 per prescription.	For insured persons: USD6 per day/maximum 28 days per year. For dependents: USD 10-USD 13.50 per day/maximum 28 days per year.	Same as for GPs.
Belgium	25%, reduced to 10% for vulnerable groups.	Same as for GPs.	Flat rate plus 1/20/30/50%; 100% for drugs on negative list.	USD5-USD6 per day, USD2-USD3 for vulnerable groups. Increased after 90 days.	
Canada	None.	None.	Discretion of Provinces.	None.	None.
Czech Republic (2000)	None.	None.	Generics covered. Non-generics reimbursed if no alternative.	None.	None.
Denmark	None, except for under 3% of the population.	None, except for under 3% of the population.	Flat rate plus: 50/70/100%.	None.	None.
Finland	There is an annual maximum fee of EUR 22 for a 12-month period. If the annual fee has not been paid, the fee is EUR 11 per visit. This fee may be collected for a maximum of three visits during the calendar year. Fee for visits outside normal opening hours is EUR 15 per visit. Fees are not collected from persons under the age of 18.	Visit to the outpatient department is EUR 22 per visit, free of charge in the psychiatric outpatient treatment unit.	SII reimburses part of the cost of medicines prescribed by the physician or dentist. SII pays 50% of all medicine costs in excess of a fixed minimum per purchase (EUR 10) or, more rarely, nearly all medicine costs (scheme members with certain specified conditions qualify for a 75% or 100% refund of costs exceeding EUR 5). All non-covered medicine costs in excess of EUR 604.72 in a year are covered by SII. Drugs administered during inpatient care are included in the daily fee.	Health centre: EUR 26 per day, EUR 12 per day in the psychiatric unit. Fees may be collected from a person under the age of 18 for only seven bed-days per calendar year. Hospital: EUR 26 per day, EUR 12 per day in the psychiatric unit. Fees may be collected from a person under the age of 18 for only 7 bed-days per calendar year. Day surgery is EUR 72 per procedure. Long-term (> 3 months) institutional care in a health centre or in a hospital: Fees according to solvency. Fees may constitute a maximum of 80% of the client's income. There must remain, for the personal use of the client, a minimum of EUR 80 per month. Fees may be collected from a person under the age of 18 for only seven bed-days per calendar year.	None.
France	30%[2]	30%[2]	0% for some drugs; 35% for most drugs, 65% for "comfort" drugs or those without proven therapeutic value.	EUR 11 per day plus 20% of total cost for first 30 days up to a ceiling of EUR 200.	40%
Germany[3] (2004)	Fee of EUR 10 per quarter covers all visits during the quarter. Preventive measures are exempt from practice fees.	Patients who are referred by one doctor to another pay no additional practice fees, as long as the referral falls within the same quarter.	Co-payment amounting to 10% of the price, but no less than EUR 5 and no more than EUR 10 per medication.	Co-payment of EUR 10 per day, limited to a maximum of 28 days in a calendar year.	None.
Greece	None.	None.	0/10/25%	USD 15	–

Table 2.2. Cost-sharing policies in public schemes for basic health coverage[1] (cont.)

Degree of cost-sharing in per cent and in USD or EUR

	General practitioner	Specialist	Drugs	Inpatient care	X-ray and pathology
Hungary (2002)	None.	Co-payment if no referral from medical doctor (except emergency).	0/10/30/50 or 100%; some drugs based on reference price system.	Co-payment for long-term care in hospitals (may be covered, depending on income level), co-payment for above-standard "hotel services" in hospitals.	None.
Iceland[4]	USD 9	USD 17 plus 40% of the rest of the cost.	0, 12.5%, 25%	None.	USD 13
Ireland[5]	None for Category I (35% of population); those in Category II pay for GP services.	As for GPs.	No charge for Category I; reimbursement for Category II of any cost over USD 21 per month.	No charge for Category I; Category II: USD 17 per day subject to a maximum of USD 166 in any 12 month period.	None for Category I.
Italy	None.	Maximum of USD 41	Free for Category I medication; 50% for Category II; both Categories I and II are free to exempted persons; 100% for Category III medication.	None.	Up to a maximum of USD 41.
Japan[6]	30% (younger than three years, 20%).	Same as for GPs	30% (younger than 3 years, 20%).	Same as for GPs	Same as for GPs (outpatient) or inpatient care.
Korea	"Outpatient fees" as follows: 30% if seen in clinic, 40% if hospital; 55% if general hospital.	"Outpatient fees" as follows: 30% if seen in clinic, 40% if hospital; 55% if general hospital.		20% of inpatient care ("hospitalization fees").	
Luxembourg	5%	5%	0% or 20%	Flat rate between EUR 10 and EUR 15	
Mexico	No cost sharing for the members of the social security schemes (these cover around half of the population). For Ministry of Health Facilities, which are open to all the population, the Ministry of Finance sets indicative rates of cost sharing that depend on household income, but the rates applied can vary among states and hospitals.				
Netherlands	None.	None.	Generics covered. Non-generics covered if no alternative.	None.	None.
New Zealand	Extra billing.	Outpatients USD 3-USD 17.	USD 2-USD 8 with stop loss.	None.	Out-patients USD 3-USD 17.
Norway	USD 11	USD 16	25% if on blue ticket, maximum USD 43 per prescription.	None.	X-ray USD 11.
Poland (1999)	None.	None.	Basic drug list: flat fee = 0.05% of min. wage; suppl. list = 30-50% of cost of drug. Patients w/ chronic disease or war veterans fully or partially reimbursed.	None.	None.
Portugal		USD 91-USD 213	0/30/60/100% depending on drug category.	USD 30	
Slovak Republic (2000)	None.	None.	Category I: fully covered. II: Same drugs as above, different manuf. partially reimbursed. III: out of pocket.	None.	None.
Spain	None.	None.	0%, 40%. Pensioners and long-term ill largely exempt.[7]	None.	None.

Table 2.2. **Cost-sharing policies in public schemes for basic health coverage**[1] (cont.)

Degree of cost-sharing in per cent and in USD or EUR

	General practitioner	Specialist	Drugs	Inpatient care	X-ray and pathology
Sweden	USD 13-USD 20 per visit. Maximum visiting fees per 12 months, USD 120 (including fees to GPs).	USD 26-USD 40 per visit. Maximum visiting fees per 12 months, USD 120 (including fees to GPs).	Patient pays 100% up to USD 120, after that, patient pays in three steps: 50%, 25% and 10% of the cost. Maximum patient fees for pharmaceuticals per 12 months USD 240.	Maximum USD 10 per day where some county councils have variations in costs, depending on age, income, etc. Local variations also with regard to maximum inpatient fees. Fees for inpatient care are not included in the high-cost protection system for outpatient care.	None.
Switzerland[8]	10%	10%	10%	CHF 10 per day (about USD7) if single.	10%
Turkey	None.	None.	10% retired; 20% active	None.	None.
United Kingdom	None.	None.	USD 9 per prescription or free with a "season ticket" of USD 130. Many persons exempt.	None.	None.
United States (2004)[9]	20% in excess of the USD 100 deductible. Also a USD 66.60 monthly premium for coverage of physician services.	20% in excess of the USD 100 deductible. Also a USD 66.60 monthly premium for coverage of physician services.	100%	USD 876 deductible first 60 hospital days; USD 219 co-payment per day for days 61-90; USD 438 per day beyond 90 days. USD 109.50 per skilled nursing facility stay day 21-100.	Same as doctors.

1. Approximate amounts in US dollars or euros, converted at nominal exchange rates. Information refers to the most recent data available, ranging from the late 1990s to the present. Some changes arising from most recent reforms may not have been included.
2. 30% of the agreed fee schedule (doctor conventionné) and more if there is overbilling. Co-payment may be less if covered by complementary insurance which normally covers part of the co-payment including the overbilling. Complementary insurance covers over 80% of the population. Vulnerable groups and long-term ill may have zero co-payment.
3. Overall co-payment ceiling per year is 2% of gross income (1% for chronically ill patients). No co-payments for those < 18 years of age.
4. Maximum for the year in the charging scheme.
5. About 40% of the population has private health insurance that generally covers general practitioner fees above a relatively high threshold, consultant/specialist fees above a certain threshold and private and semi-private accommodation. Tax relief at the marginal rate is available on unreimbursed medical expenses above a certain threshold.
6. In Japan, there is a dedicated mandatory public health system for those aged 75 and over and those aged between 65 and 74 with severe disability. From October 2002, cost sharing is 10% (20% for those with income above certain amounts).
7. Patients with chronic illness pay 10% up to maximum of 400 pesetas (USD 2.75) per prescription.
8. Plus a yearly flat rate of CHF 300 for adults, CHF 0 for children. From 1986 higher rates can be chosen up to CHF 1 500 in exchange for a lower premium. The excess of 10% pertains to the amount exceeding the flat rate but only up to a maximum amount of CHF 700 per year for an adult of CHF 350 per year for children.
9. Applies to 13% of population (elderly and disabled) who are beneficiaries of public Medicare programme. Lower deductibles if in HMOs.

Source: Information supplied by OECD member countries or obtained from official publications.

Table 2.3. **Main source of public funding for long-term care services in selected OECD countries, 2003**

	Service[1]	Main source of funding[2]	Coverage[3]
Australia	Nursing home care	General taxation	Means-tested
	Personal care at home	General taxation	Means-tested
Austria	Nursing home care	General taxation	Universal
	Personal care at home	General taxation	Universal
Canada[4]	Nursing home care	General taxation	Means-tested in most provinces
	Personal care at home	General taxation	Means-tested in most provinces
Germany	Nursing home care	Contributions	Universal
	Personal care at home	Contributions	Universal
Ireland	Nursing home care	General taxation	Means-tested
	Personal care at home	General taxation	Means-tested
Japan	Nursing home care	Contributions and general taxation	Universal
	Personal care at home	Contributions and general taxation	Universal
Korea	Nursing home care	General taxation	Means-tested
	Personal care at home	General taxation	Means-tested
Luxembourg	Nursing home care	Contributions and general taxation	Universal
	Personal care at home	Contributions and general taxation	Universal
Netherlands	Nursing home care	Contributions	Universal
	Personal care at home	Contributions	Universal
New Zealand	Nursing home care	General taxation	Means-tested
	Personal care at home	General taxation	Means-tested
Norway	Nursing home care	General taxation	Universal
	Personal care at home	General taxation	Universal
Spain	Nursing home care	General taxation	Means-tested
	Personal care at home	General taxation	Means-tested
Sweden	Nursing home care	General taxation	Universal
	Personal care at home	General taxation	Universal
United Kingdom	Nursing home care	General taxation	Means-tested[5]
	Personal care at home	General taxation	Means-tested in most areas
United States	Nursing home care	General taxation	Means-tested
	Personal care at home	General taxation	Means-tested

1. Services covered are nursing and personal care in a nursing home, and personal care in one's own home. It does not include "hotel" charges in nursing homes. Nursing care furnished in one's own home is normally covered by the acute health system in all countries.
2. General taxation may be national, regional or local. Contributions are those made to a social insurance scheme.
3. If coverage is not subject to a test of income or assets, it is shown as "universal", although there may be other restricting criteria. If coverage is subject to a test of income or assets it is shown as "means-tested".
4. Long-term care is devolved to the provinces. The table shows the situation in the majority of provinces.
5. Except in Scotland.

Source: OECD (2004b).

Some barriers to access persist

Universal health coverage, combined with low cost sharing, has proven effective in promoting equitable use of health services. Yet inequities in service use persist in some countries. These reflect factors such as the impact of user fees on lower-income groups and differences in insurance coverage across the population. The outcome can be poorer health, which further fuels economic isolation and social exclusion.

Figure 2.1. **Equity of access to physician care, 2000**

Horizontal inequity (HI) indices for probability of a doctor visit with 95% confidence intervals.

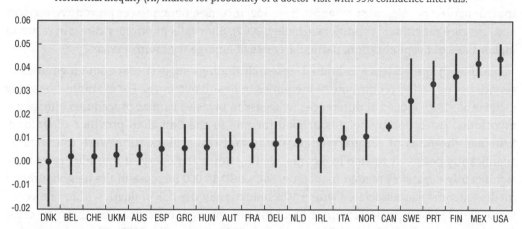

Note: The plotted points are horizontal inequity (HI) indices which summarize the inequality in the probability of at least one doctor visit (per annum) across income quintiles after need differences (variations in self reported health) have been standardised. Positive values of HI indicate inequity favouring the rich. Negative values indicate inequity favouring the poor. The "whiskers" show 95% confidence intervals. A zero or non significant value of HI indicates that the probability of a doctor visit is distributed equitably across income groups.

Source: Van Doorslaer *et al.* (2004).

New evidence on income-related equity in service use

In most OECD countries, doctor visits are distributed equitably across income groups when adjusted for need, according to an analysis of data from household surveys carried out around 2000 (Van Doorslaer *et al.*, 2004).[8] Significant inequity in doctor visits (primary and specialty care aggregated) emerged in five of 21 countries studied: Finland, Mexico, Portugal, Sweden and the United States (Figure 2.1). Such inequities are likely to spring from different root causes. For example, the pro-rich inequity found in the United States would be reduced by 30% if the insurance coverage gap were eliminated.

Like doctor visits overall, primary-care visits are equitably distributed across income groups in the majority of countries with available data. Where significant inequity appears, it is often negative, indicating a pro-poor distribution. The pattern is very different with respect to medical specialist consultations, however. In every country studied, after controlling for need differences, the rich are significantly more likely to see a specialist than are the poor, and in most countries also more frequently. This pro-rich inequity has been found to be especially large in Portugal, due to large out-of-pocket costs and unequal distribution of specialist services; in Ireland, where there are income-based differences in sources of coverage (public/private); and in Finland, because of high co-payments and privately financed delivery options.

Within several countries, differences in health care between richer and poorer regions contribute to overall income-related inequalities in secondary care. Besides Portugal, pro-rich regional differences in specialist visits are also evident in Spain, Hungary, Greece and Italy. Very often, this appears to reflect discrepancies between better-endowed regions (often the national capital area) and peripheral regions.

No clear pattern for either pro-rich or pro-poor inequity in inpatient care emerges across countries. Significant pro-poor inequity in the probability of hospital admission is found for several countries, including Australia, Canada, Switzerland and the United

States. In the United States, evidence of a pro-poor distribution of hospital admissions together with a pro-rich distribution of doctor consultations is consistent with findings that uninsured people, most of whom have low incomes, obtain fewer preventive services and less care for chronic conditions (Hadley, 2002). Shortfalls in primary care can result in higher rates of hospitalization, particularly use of emergency room services.

Although the evidence is limited, research findings suggest that some inequities in service use do, in fact, contribute to inequities in health outcomes. For example, one study (Alter *et al.*, 1999) looked at differences in access to invasive cardiac procedures after acute myocardial infarction by neighbourhood income in the Canadian province of Ontario. Whereas the rates of coronary angiography and revascularization were found to be significantly positively related to income, waiting times and one-year mortality rates were significantly negatively related to income. Each USD 10 000 increase in the neighbourhood median income was associated with a 10% reduction in the risk of death within one year.[9] Similar evidence on socio-economic inequities in coronary operations has been reported for other countries, *e.g.* Finland (Hetemaa *et al.*, 2003; Keskimäki, 2003). This suggests that differences in diagnostic and therapeutic utilization across income groups play a role in differential outcomes by income, even in a country like Canada that seems to achieve a fairly equitable distribution of care.

Mitigating the impact of patient cost-sharing on access to needed care

As part of efforts to reduce public spending or increase consumer cost-sensitivity, some OECD countries have, in recent years, introduced or increased patient cost-sharing on different types of health services.[10] New cost-sharing policies for ambulatory care or some hospital services have been introduced recently in several European countries (*e.g.* Belgium, Finland, France, Ireland, Luxembourg and Sweden) as well as in Japan. However, greater cost-sharing has mainly affected pharmaceuticals. The number of drugs not reimbursed has increased, especially so-called "lifestyle" drugs or those of uncertain therapeutic value. The degree of cost-sharing has been increased for many others.

Co-payments can have undesirable effects on access to care in some cases. In order to avoid creating financial barriers to access, the introduction of these new cost-sharing policies has generally been accompanied by measures to exempt the most vulnerable groups. Exemption can be income-based,[11] as in Italy, or tied to particular health conditions (those likely to incur high health-care costs). Under some public and private insurance arrangements, certain services (such as preventive care) are exempted from cost-sharing requirements to encourage use of such services. Some coverage also includes caps on total out-of-pocket spending to protect access to care and individual finances. Depending on design, some of these mechanisms to promote access can impose significant administrative costs on systems.

Differentiation of insurance coverage often contributes to access inequities

Private health insurance can create or exacerbate differences in access to care between populations with and without such coverage. This may reflect a country's decision to ration certain services by willingness to pay, or occur inadvertently, as a by-product of efforts to use private health insurance to meet other policy goals. In countries where waiting for certain publicly financed services is common, persons with duplicate insurance policies can obtain more timely access to these services than those with public cover alone.[12] In some of these cases, certain hospitals cater exclusively to privately insured patients and physicians may face incentives to give preferential treatment to privately financed patients. In cases where supply is tight, this can exacerbate perceived shortages of services for patients with only public cover. Those with supplemental private insurance may also obtain better access to certain goods or services not covered in public health programmes, usually luxury (*e.g.* private hospital rooms) or ancillary services, but in some cases also prescription medicines and other care of clinical importance. In the US Medicare programme for the elderly, where cost sharing is significant and prescription drugs and other services are not covered, those with additional coverage (private or public, through Medicaid) to supplement and complement Medicare have better access to care, according to measures such as cost-related delays in seeking care (Medicare Payment Advisory Commission, 2002).

Private health insurance, particularly where it is primary for some populations or supplements relatively generous public cover, need not necessarily create differential access between those with and without such coverage, however. In Germany, the United Kingdom, and Switzerland, for example, the existence of some voluntary private schemes, mainly covering additional comfort and luxury, has had only a small pro-rich contribution to otherwise fairly equitable distributions of care (Van Doorslaer *et al.*, 2004).

Policy interventions have sometimes mitigated inequities posed by differential coverage, where these were not desired. In France, voluntary purchase of private supplementary cover for co-payments had a substantial pro-rich contribution to use of specialist care services (Van Doorslaer *et al.*, 2004). But the introduction of similar public cover for the poor through the *Couverture Maladie Universelle* in 2000 brought about a significant pro-poor shift that largely compensates for this. In the Netherlands, where private health insurance is the primary source of coverage for those with high incomes, all providers treat both publicly and privately insured individuals equally, with no differential access to care by insurance status. Equity of access is facilitated by provider reimbursement limits that are applicable to both social and private insurers. Patients also have the same level of choice over the timing of care and are included on the same waiting lists.

Where differential access by insurance status is not desired, countries with private health insurance can minimise the likelihood of this through practices such as: assuring adequate coverage for the poor; establishing explicit rules to assure equity of access to care; minimising provider discretion by assigning management of waiting lists to a disinterested party; specifying and monitoring obligations of providers towards publicly insured patients; and allocating elective care on the basis of a single waiting list for both publicly and privately insured patients (OECD, 2004c).

Identifying and overcoming non-financial barriers to health care

Access to necessary health care may still vary across population groups in countries with health systems that have universal coverage and low or zero cost sharing. For example, there is often poor take-up of preventive programmes by disadvantaged groups in these countries, despite their higher risk. In Canada, for instance, the use of preventive perinatal care has been reported to be lower among mothers with lower levels of education, despite a greater risk of having low birth weight babies and a greater risk of their infants having to be hospitalised at least once during their first year. This suggests the persistence of important non-financial barriers to access, given that access to these pre-natal and post-natal services is universal and free-of-charge in Canada (Wolfson and Alvarez, 2002).

Education is an important contributor to a pro-poor distribution of doctor and dentist consultations in several countries (Van Doorslaer *et al.*, 2004). Controlling for factors such as income and health status, those with higher educations are more inclined to consult doctors and dentists in Hungary, the United States and other countries.

In the United States, evidence of inequity in the use of health services by race and ethnicity has spurred concern among policy makers. A recent study of Medicare enrolees provided strong evidence that blacks are less likely to receive recommended clinical care for a number of conditions, controlling for other factors known to be important in determining service use (Schneider *et al.*, 2002). The reasons underlying these differences in care are not yet well understood.

The United States is not alone in having such concerns. Australia, Canada and New Zealand, for instance, have concerns about equity of access for indigenous populations. The specific barriers to access might vary across countries and population groups.

Ensuring an adequate supply of health-care providers

Ensuring accessible health care requires maintaining a health workforce that is able to meet the population's need for safe, high-quality medical services. This implies an adequate number of health-care practitioners with the right qualifications, and in the right place when patients need them. However, adequacy is hard to assess, particularly if one considers that the volume of services demanded by a well-insured population may exceed the level indicated on the basis of need alone, and that some discretion is possible in the mix of skill levels used in furnishing services.

Concerns have been voiced in a number of OECD countries that a gap may be looming between demand for and supply of the services of physicians and nurses. Indeed shortages have already appeared in a number of OECD countries. Despite increasing demand for services, supply is projected to fall, or at best to grow slowly (in the absence of countermeasures) as a result of a societal trend towards reduced hours of work, physician workforce ageing, and trends towards early and partial retirement. In response to this, many countries are seeking to increase the number and the productivity of physicians and nurses in their workforces.

How many physicians are needed to ensure adequate supply of services?

The size of the physician workforce and the rate of its growth vary quite significantly across countries (Figures 2.2 and 2.3). Physician density, for example, ranges from fewer than two practising physicians per 1 000 population to double that in a number of OECD countries. Even more variation is observed in nurse density. The size, distribution and composition of practicing physicians is influenced by a number of factors, including restrictions imposed on entry into the medical profession, choice of specialty, demographic characteristics of doctors (*e.g.* age and sex), remuneration, working conditions, location of practice and migration.

There is no single answer to the question of the necessary number of physicians per capita required to ensure adequate access to care, as productivity and other factors must be taken into account. Because high physician density may give rise to unnecessary increases in service provision (so-called "supplier-induced demand"), particularly where physicians are paid on a fee-for-service basis, countries may wish to avoid oversupply so as to minimize costs.[13] On the other hand, there are signs of an inverse relationship between physician density and waiting times for elective surgery (among those countries in which waiting times are reported to be a policy concern), indicating that density levels that are too low may have a cost in terms of responsiveness or even access to care (Figure 2.4).

Figure 2.2. **Practising physicians per 1 000 population, 2000**

Figure 2.3. **Increase in number of practising physicians per 1 000 population, 1980-2000**

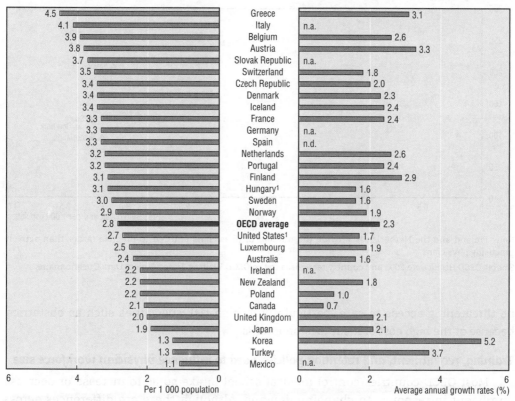

	Per 1 000 population	Average annual growth rates (%)
Greece	4.5	3.1
Italy	4.1	n.a.
Belgium	3.9	2.6
Austria	3.8	3.3
Slovak Republic	3.7	n.a.
Switzerland	3.5	1.8
Czech Republic	3.4	2.0
Denmark	3.4	2.3
Iceland	3.4	2.4
France	3.3	2.4
Germany	3.3	n.a.
Spain	3.3	n.d.
Netherlands	3.2	2.6
Portugal	3.2	2.4
Finland	3.1	2.9
Hungary[1]	3.1	1.6
Sweden	3.0	1.6
Norway	2.9	1.9
OECD average	2.8	2.3
United States[1]	2.7	1.7
Luxembourg	2.5	1.9
Australia	2.4	1.6
Ireland	2.2	n.a.
New Zealand	2.2	1.8
Poland	2.2	1.0
Canada	2.1	0.7
United Kingdom	2.0	2.1
Japan	1.9	2.1
Korea	1.3	5.2
Turkey	1.3	3.7
Mexico	1.1	n.a.

Notes: Belgium, Denmark, France, Iceland, Luxembourg and the United States include physicians working in industry, administration and research. The Czech Republic, Mexico and Norway report full time equivalents (FTE) rather than headcounts. Finland, Ireland and Netherlands provide the number of physicians entitled to practise rather than actively practising physicians. The average excludes: Germany, Ireland, Italy, Mexico, Slovak Republic and Spain.
1. 1999.

Source: OECD Health Data 2003.

Demographic and social trends influencing the supply and productivity of the physician workforces suggest the future possibility of shortages of physician services in some countries, unless steps are taken to increase productivity[14] or increase the number of physicians per head. For example, women – who represented as few as 14.3% of practising physicians in Japan up to 48.2% in the Slovak Republic in 2000 – are an increasing share of the physician workforce in most countries. If the current tendency for women to disrupt their careers during childbearing years and to work fewer hours than their male counterparts persists, average workforce productivity may drop as the share of female physicians increases. Ageing is also likely to affect future supply, potentially reducing the number of physicians in the workforce by more than 30% by 2021 in a number of countries (Simoens and Hurst, 2004). On the other hand, other countries project an increase in the number of physicians over that period.

Other factors may influence the extent and scope of physician practice in ways that may have implications for service availability. For example, policy makers in a few OECD countries – Australia, France, and the United States – are concerned that the medical professional liability system put in place to deter malpractice and compensate victims may

Figure 2.4. **Physician density and waiting times for elective surgery, 2000**

Hip replacement

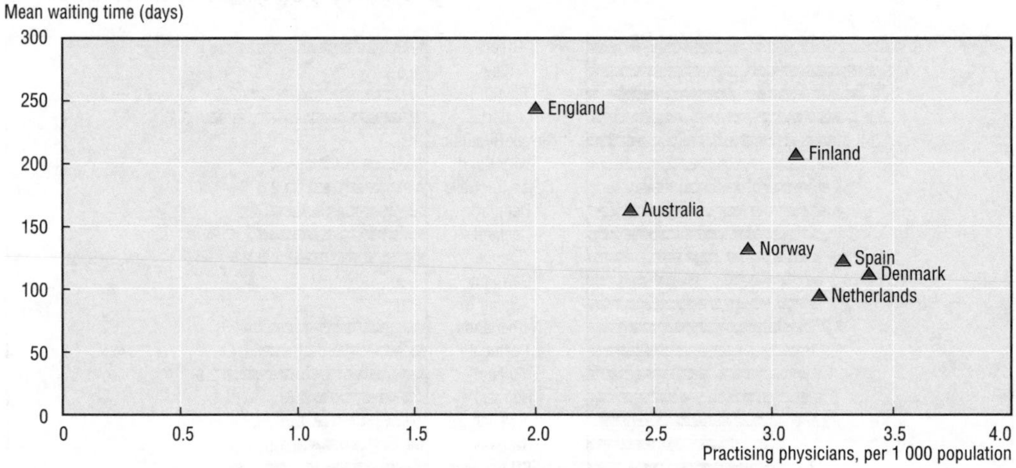

Note: Finland and the Netherlands provide the number of physicians entitled to practise rather than actively practising physicians.

Source: OECD *Health Data 2003* and country responses to the OECD Waiting Times Project Data Questionnaire.

be threatening access to care, particularly in high-risk specialties such as obstetrics, because of the high cost of insurance premiums.

Training, recruitment, and retention policies used to influence physician workforce size

Most OECD countries control medical school intake so as to increase or decrease enrolment in response to changing demand, although there are differences across countries in how tightly control is maintained. For most countries, recent graduates represented 2-3% of practising physicians in 2000 (Figure 2.5). However, Austria, Ireland and Korea had a notably larger flow of physicians joining the physician workforce in 2000, with estimates ranging from 4.5% to 9.6%.

Although countries generally favour long-term policies of national self-sufficiency to sustain their physician workforce, such policies may co-exist with short- or medium-term policies to attract physicians from abroad (see Box 2.3). Temporary migration may produce benefits in the home country through remittances and an upgrading of skills, and increase the stock of physicians in the host country. However, such considerations need to be balanced by concerns about permanent brain-drain in the home country and the quality and safety of health-care provision by migrants in the host country.[15]

Retention policies are relatively under-developed as compared with measures that aim to increase flows into the physician workforce. This may indicate that retention is not viewed as an important problem in most countries, although it may become an increasing issue as workforces age. Policies used by some countries include those to create more flexible working conditions to reduce the number of physicians that change careers and to incite physicians to defer retirement.

Responding to regional or local shortages of health-care practitioners

Many OECD countries are facing shortages of health-care practitioners in specific geographic areas. These shortages typically occur in rural areas, deprived urban areas or

Figure 2.5. **Recently graduated physicians as a percentage
of practising physicians, 2000**

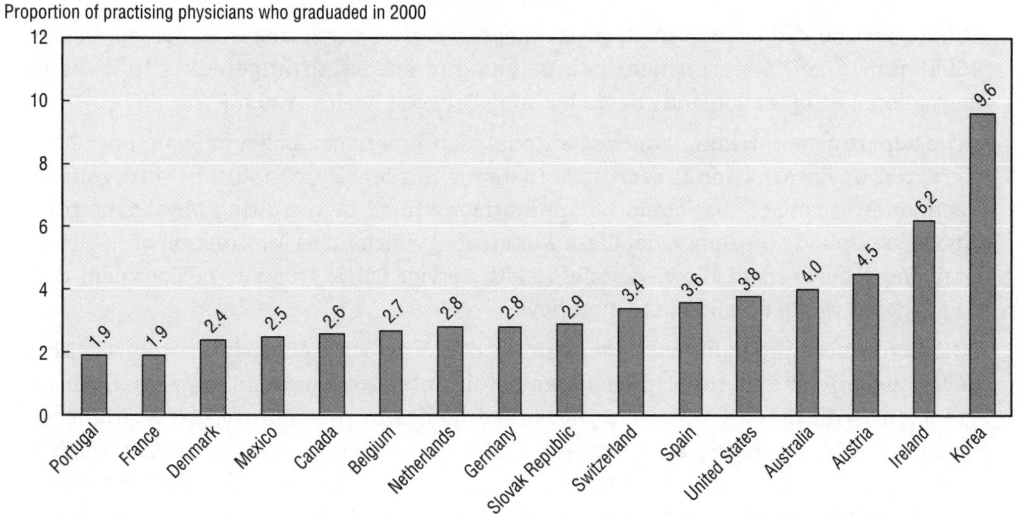

Proportion of practising physicians who graduaded in 2000

Note: Data from OECD HRHC project are based on physicians graduated who started practising during the reference year. Data from WHO Regional Office for Europe Health for All database are based on physicians graduated eligible to practise. French, Irish and Spanish data refer to 1999.

Source: Data for Australia, Canada, France, Korea, Mexico and the United States from the OECD HRHC project; data for the other countries from the WHO Regional Office for Europe Health for All database.

areas with significant indigenous populations. In response to such problems, countries have implemented policies that aim to match local supply of practitioners with population needs. Financial policies have dominated the policy landscape in Canada, although educational and regulatory policies have also been utilized to varying degrees. Regulatory policies have been predominant in Norway. New Zealand and the United Kingdom have used a combination of both policies. Policies relating to the education of physicians have been used relatively less, except in Australia, Japan, and the United States.

Financial incentives have been used to compensate for the additional demands associated with practising in rural areas and the limited economic viability of practising in such areas due to the sparse population base. Regionally differentiated remuneration to physicians for patients from rural or deprived areas increases payments relative to those for patients from other areas. Other policies that offer practice establishment grants, travel grants, relocation grants and financial support of locums seem to have had some success in increasing the number of physicians practising in targeted areas. However, it is unclear whether such policies are more or less costly than educational or regulatory approaches.

Educational initiatives that attract medical students who came from a rural background and prioritise training programmes that emphasise the rural component of the curriculum have had some success. The Physician Shortage Area Program in the United States, for instance, consists of a selective admission policy for students of rural origin, financial aid, a family medicine programme and selection of rural practice sites. Such multi-faceted programmes have been successful in recruiting physicians to rural areas as well as retaining them. On the other hand, policies that provide scholarships to medical students in return for a commitment to practice in rural areas for a number of years can be less effective because students sometimes bought their way out of their service

Box 2.3. **The UK experience with policies stimulating immigration of physicians**

Strategies adopted by the British government to attract physicians from abroad include global and targeted recruitment campaigns and special arrangements that foster international co-operation and shared learning between health systems.

The Department of Health launched a global recruitment campaign in September 2001. It created an international recruitment team to identify consultant and general practitioner vacancies that could be appropriately filled by recruiting physicians from outside the United Kingdom. A database was created which holds information of sufficient detail and robustness to allow National Health Service (NHS) Trusts to be confident that the applicant would be suitable to interview.

UK recruitment programmes target certain countries with physician surpluses. This process usually entails the establishment of an inter-governmental agreement or an agreement with the appropriate professional bodies in the country. For example, in November 2000 the United Kingdom and Spain made such an agreement. Although it initially applied to the migration of nurses, the agreement has now been extended to cover the recruitment of specialists and general practitioners. As part of the recruitment package, each Spanish recruit is offered individual language courses and participation in an induction programme covering information about their chosen speciality, the National Health Service, the roles and responsibilities of their profession, and general information about living in the United Kingdom and British culture. The international recruitment team is working with other countries with perceived surpluses such as Switzerland, Austria, Italy, Greece, Bulgaria and India.

Special arrangements foster international co-operation and promote the NHS abroad by shared learning between health systems. An International Fellowship Programme was launched in 2002 to attract experienced specialists from abroad to selected posts in the NHS for periods of one to two years. It targets specialties that need to grow in order to fulfil the NHS plan and those with perceived shortages.

commitment and few students opt to remain in rural areas after their required period of service. In Canada, northern medical schools have recently been established to enhance educational opportunities for individuals from northern, and typically rural, areas.

Regulatory policies that restrict practice location have also had some success. For instance, an English policy of considering all general practitioner applications to practise in light of existing physician density, rurality, and deprivation seems to have resulted in a reasonably equitable distribution of services (Maynard and Walker, 1997). Some OECD countries have also considered policies that make immigration or remuneration conditional on practice location. More work needs to be done to determine the feasibility and cost-effectiveness of other regulatory policies, such as the substitution of nurse practitioners and registered nurses for general practitioners, and the use of new technologies such as telemedicine in rural and deprived urban areas.

There is some evidence that the effectiveness of policies focusing on the physician or nurse can be further enhanced by supporting occupational opportunities for spouses and partners, education of children and accommodation (Kamien, 1998; Rabinowitz et al., 1999). To address the problem fully, however, such policies may need to be accompanied by initiatives that enhance the economic and social viability of local communities in rural and deprived urban areas.

Addressing the nurse shortage

There are increasing concerns about nurse shortages in many OECD countries, particularly in Canada, Norway, the United Kingdom and the United States. Demand for nursing services has been increasing due to ageing populations, greater consumer activism and increasing reliance on medical technologies. At the same time, supply has failed to keep pace because of a variety of factors, including fewer younger people entering the workforce, a greater range of professional opportunities, a perception that nursing is undervalued, and negative perceptions of nurse working conditions. Nursing shortages are an important policy concern in part because numerous studies have found an association between higher nurse staffing ratios and reduced patient mortality, lower risk of medical complications, and other desired outcomes. Nursing shortages are expected to worsen as the current workforce ages.

To address nurse shortages, policy makers have supported enrolments into nursing school, stimulated immigration of foreign(-trained) nurses. Other prospective policies include increasing nurse pay, improving working conditions and improving nurse education and training programmes. Information on the effectiveness of each of these strategies in alleviating nurse shortages is limited, and there is none on their effectiveness in comparison with each other, nor on their costs.

Efforts to increase nursing school intake have been inhibited by a variety of factors: the costs of funding additional capacity in public nursing schools; the perceived decline in the appeal of the nursing profession and size of cohorts of young people in the population; the lead time in producing fully-trained nurses; faculty shortages; and reform of training programmes to account for trends such as nurses treating more patients, making more use of technology, and being accountable for higher levels of quality of care. On the other hand, advertising and recruitment campaigns in Australia, Ireland, the United Kingdom and the United States designed to attract the interest of young people into nursing and show them what it is like to work as a nurse seem to have increased enrolments in nursing schools in these countries.

OECD countries have tried to increase the stock of practising nurses through international nurse recruitment; for example, by improving regulatory and certification processes to assist nurses in obtaining registration more easily. However, this may create a tension with the need to maintain standards, with concerns being raised in Greece, for example, about the qualifications and linguistic skills of foreign nurses and the quality of health care they provide. Alternatively, countries such as Australia have fast-tracked visa or work permit applications of foreign nurses. Some countries have adopted policies of active and targeted international recruitment of nurses. Norway, for instance, has regulated international recruitment through government-to-government agreements and has assigned responsibility for attracting a limited number of foreign nurses to a single government agency. This approach allows the government to control migration flows and balance concerns about permanent brain-drain in the home country with the need to cut nursing shortages in the host country.

Pay raises can be used to influence the extent to which trained nurses participate in the workforce. However, supply elasticities for nurses have been found to be low in the United

Kingdom and the United States, largely due to the high share of registered nurses who are already participating in the workforce. This implies that large wage increases would be required to have a noticeable impact on supply (Antonazzo *et al.*, 2003; Shields, 2003).

Evidence of nurse dissatisfaction with working conditions contributing to low morale, burn-out, turnover, work-related injuries and absenteeism suggests that countries may be able to raise nurse productivity by improving working conditions. Evidence on which workplace strategies create and maintain a work environment that attracts, retains and maximises productivity of nurses is only emerging. One interesting approach is the "Magnet Nursing Services Recognition Program", which was set up in the United States in the early 1990s to recognize hospitals with features shown to promote and sustain professional nursing practice.

Recent evidence that hospitals with a higher proportion of registered nurses exhibit improved nurse retention and lower patient mortality (Aiken *et al.*, 2003) suggests that there may be a trade-off between the number of nurses and the education of nurses in addressing nurse shortages, *i.e.* nurse shortages may be resolved by employing fewer nurses, but raising the proportion of nurses who are registered.

Recognizing that adequate staffing levels are often a prerequisite for creating attractive working conditions, some countries have implemented minimum ratios of nurses to patients. California proposed legislated nurse-patient ratios in January 2002 to take effect in 2003 and 2004, as has the state of Victoria, Australia. Since implementing its minimum staffing legislation, the Victoria government claims that 2 650 nurses who had not been working in nursing have re-entered the workforce and that demand for places in nursing schools has increased by 25.5%. In the United States, the experience of individual hospitals suggests that minimum staffing ratios are successful in reducing nurse turnover, although that sometimes came at the expense of other hospitals in the area (Lafer *et al.*, 2003). However, more evidence is needed about whether savings arising from reduced nurse turnover and shorter patient stays compensate increased costs of higher staffing levels. The implications of higher staffing levels on nurse productivity also need to be considered.

Assuring the availability of an appropriate mix of long-term care services

Inadequate institutional care capacity is seen as problematic in some countries. Australia, the United Kingdom, the United States, and some other countries face localised shortages of nursing home-beds, reflecting local housing and labour cost issues. In the case of Australia, the shortage may reflect a transition period following policy decisions that favour development of home care. Other countries, including Japan and Spain, have more widespread shortages which, in the case of Japan, may be addressed by current rapid growth in supply. In Germany, Japan, and elsewhere, there has been an increase over the past decade in the number of long-term care beds per 1 000 population aged 65 and over, which can be attributed at least partly to enhanced coverage by publicly funded programmes of long-term care in institutions.

Nevertheless, most OECD countries now have an adequate capacity to meet demand for long-term care furnished in institutions. It is no longer seen as adequate, however, that institutionalisation should be only choice available to meet long-term care needs, particularly given survey evidence showing that most people prefer to receive care at home whenever possible. Therefore, a policy goal in many OECD countries has been to shift the provision of long-term care from institutions towards community-based care. A number of

OECD countries (*e.g.* Luxembourg, the Netherlands and Norway) have seen a decline in the number of long-term care beds relative to the size of the older population, while in a number of others (*e.g.* Austria, New Zealand and the United Kingdom), this ratio has remained broadly stable even though the number of very old people within the 65+ age group continues to rise (OECD, 2004b).

In many countries, home-based care is the predominant form of long-term care received by elderly persons, who represent the majority of all long-term care recipients in OECD countries[16] (Figure 2.6). The objective is to allow the elderly to live independently for a longer time either in their own homes or in special housing arrangements adapted to their needs. Countries are focusing on the extension of services to the home setting and support for family caregivers who provide such services in the informal sector. Nevertheless, ensuring adequate supply of caregivers in the formal sector is an important current policy priority, which will grow as populations (and family caregivers) age.

Figure 2.6. **Long-term care service use among the elderly in selected OECD countries, 2000**

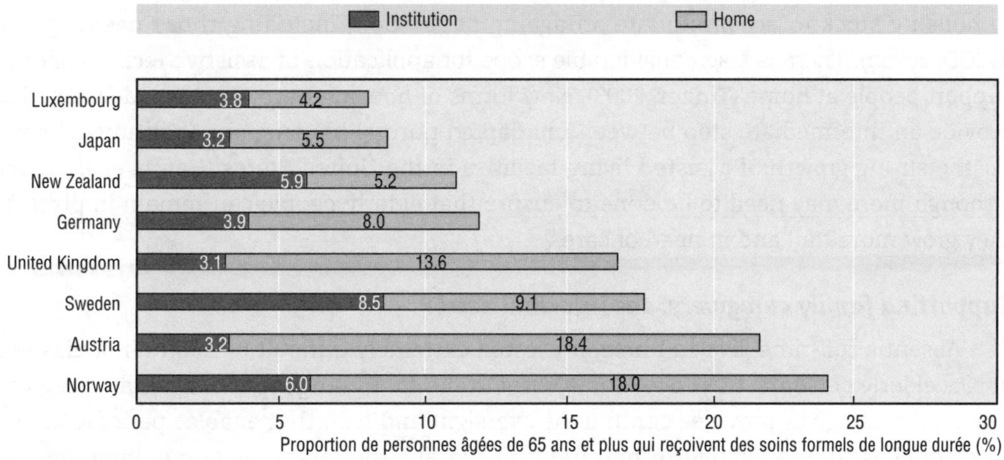

Note: Estimates are of persons receiving care in nursing homes (institutions) and of people receiving home-care allowances or services.

Source: OECD Long-Term Care Study.

Extending long-term care services to the home setting

Many countries have attempted to multiply the number of home-based options for long-term care that are available. For example, local government is mandated in the United Kingdom to increase the supply of intensive home care packages. It is also policy to consider home-based options first in many other countries. Interest in extending supply reflects both choice and cost considerations, in that institutional care can be relatively expensive. A number of schemes employ a cap on the cost per individual using home-based care that is related to the cost of a nursing home place, in effect putting a limit on the preference for home-based care.

Australia, the United Kingdom and a number of other countries have shown that it is possible to extend the boundaries of what was previously thought possible in maintaining disabled elderly people at home. Some counties have found that appropriately-targeted home care can be provided at lower cost than institutional care and can play a part in restraining acute hospital costs.[17] However, as supplying such care to all those who may be at some risk of institutionalisation would be very expensive, Sweden, the United Kingdom and the United States, among other countries, have developed a more targeted approach to home care that focuses on the more disabled elderly (OECD, 2004b).

In Australia, Germany and elsewhere the expansion of public programmes covering long-term care services has resulted in a strong growth of supply in the home-care sector, in particular. In some cases, both the public and private sector has contributed to this growth. In at least one case (Germany) the policy of increasing public funding for home care was coupled with an explicit policy to enable growth of an internally competing private provider segment rather than increasing the number of additional public providers. Countries with a traditionally high investment in institutional, public long-term care (e.g. the Netherlands, Norway, Sweden) have also greatly increased home-based alternatives for more disabled elderly people.

Increasing the provision of long-term care services at home requires inputs from several service sectors and good co-ordination of the different elements necessary to maintain older people at home, including housing, social services, visiting acute care, and other services such as shopping or household maintenance. Improvements will be needed to housing stock to accommodate an ageing population, including those needing care (OECD, 2003a). There is also considerable scope for application of assistive technologies to support people at home (Tinker, 2003). New forms of housing have also been developed to provide an intermediate step between unadapted normal housing and institutional care, e.g. the strong growth of assisted living facilities in the United States (Hawes et al., 2003), although more may need to be done to ensure that elderly people can remain in place as they grow more frail and in need of care.

Supporting family caregivers: the informal sector

Absent a full-time, live-in nurse, it is often extremely difficult to maintain a disabled or sick elderly person in their own home without the continuing input of a family caregiver. The family caregiver provides continuous oversight and help that enables periodic home-care services to be effective in maintaining the elderly person at home. Providing an adequate choice of care setting has thus come to be seen to require support of the family caregiver. Many new services, such as call-out services or respite care, have been developed specifically with family caregivers in mind.

In some countries it is no longer considered appropriate to regard family care as a "free good" and there is recognition that the caregiver needs support. These countries have adapted social protection and employment mechanisms to enable potential family caregivers of working age, where they wish and are able to do so, to combine work and caring responsibilities. This entails some mix of income support to help replace current earnings, pension credits to maintain future income prospects in retirement, and flexibility in employment terms. For example, Australia and the United Kingdom pay a caregiver pension similar to benefits for other people unable to work, in cases where the caregiver is of working age. Austria has an extensive system of care allowances, under which the recipient can use the cash benefit to compensate family caregivers. Germany's long-term care insurance has an option whereby the recipient can choose to take all or part of the benefit in cash to compensate a family caregiver. In some countries, a family caregiver may be employed as social services staff where this is considered to be the best way to provide care (e.g. in remote areas in Nordic countries).

Whether such policies are more efficient than subsidising more formal assistance is unclear, particularly given that women, who have long served as most informal caregivers, are increasingly educated and trained for the paid workforce. Most countries do not now pay family caregivers for services which traditionally have been provided with no charge on public funds, leaving any compensation to be decided within the family. Given that projections of informal care suggest that in the future, fewer caregivers will be of working age, policy makers' focus will likely continue to be on provision of services to support caregivers over retirement age, rather than on reimbursement of absences from the labour market.

Growing the long-term care workforce: the formal sector

Attracting and retaining a sufficient number of adequately trained and qualified staff to provide paid long-term care in home-based settings and institutions is the most frequently quoted concern in member countries with respect to long-term care services (OECD, 2004b). This concern is not new, but it has become of increasing importance in many countries. The long-term care sector is notorious for high turnover of staff and all countries have reported shortages in qualified nursing staff. In competition with other parts of health care, long-term care might find it even more difficult to attract sufficient numbers of adequately trained staff.

Most OECD countries project need for a larger long-term care workforce to supply services in the future. Long-term care staff are generally lower paid and receive less training than other health-care staff, and are overwhelmingly female. As the ratio of working-age to older people diminishes, lower-paid long-term care work may have greater difficulty in recruitment and retention. Strategies to attract and retain sufficient workforce in this field include offering better training and working conditions, and higher salaries (a strategy followed in some countries, e.g. Sweden), which ultimately could add to the increasing cost pressure of long-term care services.

Possibilities to substitute technology for personnel in care institutions – by keeping watch electronically on dementia patients to make sure they do not wander off, for example – seem limited, although there may be greater opportunities to use technology to enable less-dependent older people to be cared for at a distance in their own homes (Cowan and Turner-Smith, 1998).

Access to new health-related technologies

Health policy makers aim to foster timely access to new pharmaceuticals, medical devices, and other innovations, and to ensure that such innovations are safe, effective and efficient. Timely decision-making by public and private providers, payers and coverage schemes can be a difficult prospect, given the rapid pace of technological change in health care.[18]

Explaining cross-country differences in technology adoption and diffusion

Given different decision outcomes, economic incentives, and other factors, health-related technologies are adopted and diffused according to quite different patterns across the OECD (see Box 2.4). Cross-country differences in technology adoption, diffusion and use stem from a variety of factors, including explicit public decisions regarding coverage, payment, or pricing, as well as different economic incentives and administrative controls faced by practitioners, hospitals, technology manufacturers, and patients. OECD research on the diffusion of certain health technologies used in the treatment of ageing-related

Box 2.4. **Cross-country differences in the rate of adoption and diffusion of health technologies**

Studies have documented significant differences across countries in the rate of adoption and patterns of diffusion of health-related technologies. For example, a study comparing care for heart attack patients in 17 countries over the past decade (TECH Research Network, 2001) showed that, while treatment in all countries has become more intensive in the use of medications and cardiac procedures, the United States had a pattern of early adoption of new technologies and fast diffusion. Based on more limited evidence, Japan and possibly France also shared this pattern of technology use for heart attack care. By contrast, other countries showed either a late start/fast growth pattern of technological diffusion (Australia, Belgium and most Canadian provinces) or a late start/slow growth pattern (the United Kingdom, Scandinavian countries and Ontario). The patterns of diffusion for new, very high-cost drugs were similar to those for intensive procedures, but no such patterns were observed for low-cost, easy-to-use medications.

Diffusion of imaging technology provides another illustration of significant cross-country differences. On average across countries, the number of MRI (magnetic resonance imaging) scanners per capita more than tripled during the 1990s, rising from 1.7 per million population in 1990 to 6.5 in 2000 (the median was 4.7 MRI per million population in 2000). The number of CT (computed tomography) scanners also increased, albeit more moderately, from an average of 10.1 per million population in 1990 to 17.7 in 2000 (with a median of 12.1 per million in 2000). In 2000, Japan had, by far, the highest number of CT and MRI scanners per capita,[1] with 84 CT scanners per million population and 23 MRI units. The rapid increase in the number of MRI scanners in Japan has been attributed at least partly to the lack of any formal assessment of efficiency or effectiveness before making decisions to purchase MRI units (Hisashige, 1992). European countries like Switzerland, Finland, Austria and Iceland also have a relatively high number of MRI and CT scanners. At the other end of the scale, Mexico and Poland report the lowest number of CT (2 and 0.4, respectively) and MRI (0.3 and 0.4, respectively) scanners per capita.

The number of scanners provides an indication of the overall availability of such equipment, but does not indicate to what extent the equipment is used. A study comparing the use of diagnostic tests in hospitals in Canada and the United States found that American patients received many more CT and MRI tests than Canadians, a result that held even for hospitals with similar availability of machines. Much of the difference in test use was explained by the more intensive use of available machines for the elderly in the United States than in Canada (Katz *et al.*, 1996).

1. It should be noted that the figures for the United States underestimate considerably the real number of CT and MRI units in that country, because they refer to the number of hospitals reporting that they have at least one scanner rather than the total number of scanners in hospitals and in other locations (*e.g.* specialised clinics).

diseases found that demand-side constraints, such as out-of-pocket payments, had little impact on utilisation of certain treatments for heart disease, breast cancer, and stroke. On the other hand, supply-side constraints – in particular, technology regulation and payment methods for hospitals and physicians – appear to have had a noticeable effect on treatment patterns for these conditions (Moïse, 2003).

Making technology adoption and diffusion decisions under uncertainty

Those making decisions about the uptake and diffusion of new technologies often must act in the face of considerable uncertainty. The evidence that is needed to make informed decisions may not be available, especially when a technology is at a very early stage of development. Although there are no easy answers, there are ways to improve decision-making under these circumstances.

Decision makers in a growing number of countries are authorised to approve a technology on a conditional basis, limiting technology diffusion based on geography, time and/or patient groups.[19] This allows for limited access to a technology on a trial basis to enable the gathering of information about the technology. At the same time, it minimises many of the risks associated with widespread diffusion of a technology of uncertain value. However, successful use of conditional approval depends on the capacity for decision-makers to withdraw support for a technology if it is found to be relatively ineffective or inefficient.

Early identification programmes, also known as horizon scanning, may also be helpful to improve decision-making with respect to technologies. Horizon scanning can provide important information for decision makers on the emergence of new technologies and identification of available evidence and gaps. Such programmes have been successfully launched in several countries, including Canada, the Netherlands, and the United Kingdom, as well as internationally, through the EuroScan Network.[20]

Conditional approval and early identification programmes may not suffice to address the challenges presented by some of the most important emerging, health-related technologies, however (see Box 2.5). Both the processes and the type of information sought for decision-making will need to be modified to take into account the special challenges these technologies present.

Approaches for assuring adequate and equitable access: summary of findings

Ensuring comprehensive coverage of core services and minimising financial and other barriers to access has proven effective in promoting equitable use of health services. Yet inequities persist in some countries and there is evidence that these contribute to inferior health status, feeding thereby into continued economic isolation and social exclusion. Other inequities, such as differences in timeliness of service or other differences resulting from differential insurance coverage across the population may or may not be considered inappropriate.

Given extensive government intervention and failures in markets for health-care services, there is much yet to learn as to which approaches are most effective in ensuring an adequate supply of health-care providers and services. What is considered adequate will vary across systems, reflecting factors such as need, demand and productivity. A range of approaches has proven more or less effective in redressing shortages of health-care providers, where these arise, but averting shortages and surpluses is a preferable solution, though elusive.

Deficits are widespread in the availability of support services for informal care giving at home, even though it is widely recognised that outcomes and satisfaction are superior in a home-based setting. Efforts to support home-based care and informal caregivers have shown that these have helped enable a greater number of older persons to stay in their own homes and to live an independent life.

Policy makers face challenges in ensuring prompt and adequate access to new and emerging health technologies while managing communal resources appropriately. Countries differ greatly in how decisions regarding adoption of new heath-related

Box 2.5. **Decision-making challenges posed by tomorrow's technologies**

Emerging technologies, such as biomedicines, are likely to present particularly difficult challenges for decision-makers. It has been estimated that by 2015 the market share of genome-based drugs, which are likely to have a fundamental impact on the very way in which disease is understood and treated, will grow to 40% of the total pharmaceutical market (Tollman et al., 2001).[1] Hence, decisions on the adoption and application of these technologies can be expected to have far-reaching economic, clinical and social consequences.

Many of the potential new technologies, such as the use of stem cells and gene therapy, present formidable challenges to decision makers. The technologies tend to be more personalised to individual situations, making generalisations difficult. They also touch on human values such as privacy and confidentiality, as well as complex ethical questions relating to the start and end of life and the use of information. Further, public and media attention to medical biotechnologies is sometimes intense.

Biomedicine may challenge current methodologies for evaluating the benefits of new technologies. For example, analysing the cost-effectiveness of genetic testing has been problematic, in part because of the difficulty in assessing the value of the information provided through such tests. Furthermore, conditional approval may not be appropriate for value-laden technologies because of the widespread implications that the first decision has for subsequent decisions, including research and development.

More often, however, especially with value-laden, controversial or innovative medical techniques, decisions about research, adoption and uptake are required at increasingly earlier stages. But often such decisions are delayed because decision makers do not have the appropriate processes in place and information available to enable sound policy making. More work at the international level could provide policy makers with useful tools for addressing these challenges.

1. Tissue engineering, for example, is expected to grow from a market volume of USD 232 million in 2000 to more than USD 1 billion by 2007 (Frost and Sullivan, 2001).

technology are made, and these in turn reflect diffusion. Some technologies pose particular challenges that can make decision-making particularly difficult; however, approaches such as conditional approval and early identification programmes can help decision makers make appropriate decisions when faced with uncertainty.

Notes

1. *Public financing* for coverage comes mainly through taxation or income-related payroll taxes, including social security contributions.

2. *Private health insurance* is coverage financed mainly through private non-income related payments (premiums) made to an insuring entity. This coverage guarantee is usually set forth in a contract between a private party and the insurer that spells out the terms and conditions for payment or reimbursement of services. The insurer assumes much or all of the risk for paying for the contractually specified services.

3. So-called Medigap insurance, which supplements and complements public Medicare coverage for the elderly and disabled, plays a similar role in the United States.

4. In Australia, the population covered declined steadily since the mid-1980s and throughout the 1990s due to the establishment of universal public insurance in 1984 and a process of adverse selection in the market. Government policies to support private cover beginning in 2000 have increased levels of coverage to over 40%. In Ireland, a booming economy and the increasing

provision of private health insurance as a work-related benefit are responsible for uninterrupted growth in coverage from 22% in 1979 to 48% in 2002, despite an expansion in the generosity of public cover. In other OECD countries, such as the Netherlands, France and the United States, private coverage has remained fairly stable.

5. Segmentation of private health insurance markets reduces the extent to which health-care costs are shared across persons of different risks and can cause problems of affordability for high-risk persons.

6. All provinces in Canada provide prescription drug coverage to seniors and social assistance recipients (Canadian Institute for Health Information, 2003). Some Canadian provinces provide coverage for certain other populations (*e.g.* those persons prescribed certain high-cost drugs).

7. Recently enacted US legislation added a new prescription drug coverage benefit for Medicare beneficiaries. Until this benefit takes effect, a discount drug programme is intended to help reduce the costs of prescription drugs for beneficiaries without supplemental insurance coverage.

8. All of the findings pertaining to equity of service use discussed in this section are drawn from Van Doorslaer *et al.* (2004), unless otherwise attributed.

9. More recently, the same research team (Alter *et al.*, 2004) found that socioeconomic status was not significantly associated with mortality at one year following hospitalization for myocardial infarction, despite the fact that more affluent or better educated patients were morelikely to undergo coronary angiography,receive cardiac rehabilitation,or be followed up by a cardiologist.

10. Cost sharing takes the form of **co-payments**, or fixed amounts required of patients using care (also known as user fees); **co-insurance**, a fixed percentage of costs to be borne by patients; and **deductibles**, set amounts patients must pay out of pocket before insurance coverage kicks in.

11. This is consistent with research findings reviewed in the context of an assessment of the recent health-system reform experience in OECD countries, which show that the impact of cost sharing on demand is higher for low-income households (Docteur and Oxley, 2003).

12. This is the case, for example, in Australia, Ireland, Spain and the United Kingdom.

13. Although there is no conclusive evidence regarding the incidence and extent of supplier-induced demand, physicians do have considerable discretion over practice patterns, which are influenced by, amongst other things, ethical constraints, practice protocols, amount of available time and views on their appropriate level of income.

14. See discussion of prospects for increasing physician productivity in Chapter 5.

15. For discussion of mobility of highly skilled health professionals in the case of South Africa, see OECD (2003f).

16. Across OECD countries for which estimates are available, elderly people represent about 80% of home-care recipients and about 90% of the institutional-care recipients (OECD, 2004b).

17. This has been the case in Canada (see Hollander and Chappell, 2002) and in the United Kingdom (see Davies and Fernandez, 2003).

18. For example, in the year 2002, the US Food and Drug Administration (FDA) approved some 78 new drug applications and 152 expanded indications. The FDA also approved 34 major new biological agents and 34 biotech agents that were substantially equivalent to existing products, and 4 949 new or modified devices (including 41 major new devices). This is in addition to many advances in clinical procedures, such as lung volume reduction surgery, which were not related to new products and, therefore, not reflected in the activities of the FDA (Gelijns *et al.*, 2004).

19. In Switzerland, for example, tests for infectious diseases such as hepatitis C were recently granted a five-year approval. During this time, Swiss regulators will seek additional data to resolve key uncertainties. Statistical standards have been agreed and will provide information to the regulators and also provide important R&D information to manufacturers of the tests.

20. The Euroscan network is comprised of twelve members, primarily technology assessment agencies, in ten countries, including two outside of Europe (Canada and Israel). It aims to establish a network to evaluate and exchange information on new and changing technologies, develop the sources of information used to identify new and emerging technologies, develop applied methods for early assessment, and disseminate information on early identification and assessment activities.

ISBN 92-64-01555-8
Towards High-Performing Health Systems
© OECD 2004

Chapter 3

Satisfied patients and consumers: the quest for greater responsiveness

Assuring that patients are satisfied with their care and with the system in which they obtain it is an increasingly important policy objective in OECD countries (Kalisch *et al.*, 1998). This is likely to reflect evidence of significant dissatisfaction with health systems and specific aspects of the systems. For example, in the European Union, the share of persons who report they are "very dissatisfied" with their health-care system was recently found to range between 2 and 34%, with a cross-country average of 13% (European Commission, 2001). A 2001 survey of five countries – Australia, Canada, New Zealand, the United Kingdom, and the United States – found that the vast majority of those surveyed agreed with the statement that "fundamental changes" to their health system were required or the system needed to be "rebuilt completely"(Blendon *et al.*, 2002). In the same study, however, as in others, the findings on satisfaction with overall health-system performance contrast with those revealing that the majority of individuals in each country did not report problems with their own personal experience with health care according to most measures.

Satisfaction with care and with health and long-term care systems is a function of the experiences and perceptions of individual patients and consumers. Individual judgements, in turn, are influenced by many of the same factors as policy makers use to assess system performance: perceived quality of care[1] and quality of interaction with health-care professionals and caregivers; extent of choice among providers, insurers, and treatments; affordability; fair and equitable treatment; and perceived accessibility of care, implying the timely local availability of basic services and opportunity to benefit from the latest medical advances.

Health systems have a great frontier for improvement in meeting the expectations and preferences of patients and consumers of health and long-term care. OECD work has identified policies that reduce waiting times for elective surgery and that better meet the desires of long-term care recipients, two major sources of dissatisfaction in OECD countries, and has considered how offering choice of health coverage can result in a more responsive health system.

Policies to address excessive waiting times for elective surgery

Waiting times for elective surgery (see Box 3.1) are considered problematic where they are associated with consumer dissatisfaction and a sense that the health-care system is not responsive. In such cases, waiting times can be reduced through supply-side or demand-side policies (Hurst and Siciliani, 2003). They may also be reduced by policies aimed directly at waiting times, which can affect both demand and supply at the same time.

Supply-side policies have been used in all countries with waiting-times problems on various occasions; these include expanding capacity by increasing the number of surgical staff and beds in public surgical units or by contracting for additional capacity in the private units, in line with expenditure on surgery. Doing so will raise costs *pro rata* to volume. Alternatively, productivity can be increased by linking the remuneration of doctors and hospitals with the activity performed. It may be possible to combine such policies with only modest increases in capacity and expenditure if budgetary and fee-setting discipline

Box 3.1. **Why are there excessive waiting times for elective surgery in some OECD countries?**

In at least a dozen OECD countries,[1] elective surgery candidates generally wait for some weeks or months before obtaining surgery. On the other hand, in at least eight OECD countries,[2] waiting times appear to be negligible.

Compared with the group of countries with documented waiting times, those without have higher average per capita health spending in total, in the public sector, and in the private sector. The lowest-spending countries have the longest waiting times and the highest-spending countries have no waiting times. However, one high-spending country (Norway) also reports relatively long waiting times and one low-spending country has no waiting times (Japan). Of the mid-level spending countries, four report waiting times and three do not. Low availability of acute-care beds is significantly associated with the presence of waiting times. Fee-for-service remuneration for specialists, as opposed to salaried remuneration, is negatively associated with the presence of waiting times, as is activity-based funding for hospitals.

Among the group of countries with waiting times, physician density has the most significant negative association with waiting times. Econometric estimates suggest that a marginal increase of 0.1 practising physicians and specialists per 1 000 population is associated, respectively, with a marginal reduction of mean waiting times of 8.3 and 6.4 days (at the sample mean) and a marginal reduction of median waiting times of 7.6 and 8.9 days.

1. Australia, Canada, Denmark, Finland, Ireland, Italy, Netherlands, New Zealand, Norway, Spain, Sweden and United Kingdom.
2. Austria, Belgium, France, Germany, Japan, Luxembourg, Switzerland and the United States.

Source: Siciliani and Hurst (2003).

is maintained; in other words, if some of the productivity gains are passed on in the form of lower prices per procedure. Productivity may also be enhanced by fostering day-surgery.

Demand-side policies, such as raising the clinical threshold for admitting patients to waiting lists, may be warranted if publicly funded surgeries are being provided in cases where costs exceed benefits. Such policies could increase the value of public spending on surgery. To the extent that demand-side policies prevent inappropriate additions to waiting lists and give patients certainty of eligibility for treatment, they can raise welfare. Yet dissatisfaction among prospective patients may be an issue unless privately financed surgery can be readily obtained by those individuals for who want it. Otherwise, there is a risk of merely disguising existing demand for surgery by replacing visible waiting on the waiting list with less visible "waiting to join the waiting list".

Alternatively, policies may be adopted to encourage private health insurance purchase, with the aim of diverting demand from public care to private care. However, when there is generous coverage through publicly financed schemes – more specifically, the offer of free or almost free elective surgery after a wait – the take-up for private health insurance (or out-of-pocket payment for surgery) is, with some exceptions (*e.g.* Australia and Ireland), modest.[2] This is consistent with evidence suggesting that the willingness to pay for reductions in public queuing for elective surgery is quite low.[3] Perhaps in part because of low take-up, private health insurance has not significantly reduced waiting times in OECD countries where these are considered a problem, although it has helped to finance increases in service capacity and supply in Australia.

Policies aimed directly at waiting times include imposing maximum waiting time targets (as has been done in Denmark, Italy, the Netherlands, Norway, Spain, Sweden and the United Kingdom) and providing financial incentives to surgeons or hospitals for reducing waiting times (as has been done in Spain). Maximum waiting time targets have been used successfully to eliminate very long waiting in England but appear to have had no effect on the average waiting time of all those treated. Moreover, accelerating the treatment of patients waiting longest clashes with clinical prioritisation, as those waiting longest are not necessarily those whose condition is the most severe.

Despite a number of successful initiatives to reduce waiting times, solving this problem is not simple. A common experience in addressing waiting times is to take measures aimed at increasing activity, only to find that after a brief period, demand has increased and waiting times have reverted to levels similar to those before the introduction of the measures. For example, during the 1990s, England succeeded only in stabilising the average waiting time of those admitted for 11 major elective procedures, despite a 64% rise in rates of such procedures over the course of the decade. In England as elsewhere, demand for surgery has been rising rapidly because of technological change. Moreover, demand responds positively to reductions in waiting times, as it would to reductions in price.

Long-term care that better meets the preferences and expectations of patients and caregivers

Long-term care has long been a source of dissatisfaction for both patients and caregivers. The past decade has seen much activity designed to improve the responsiveness of long-term care systems across the OECD.

Improving the institutional care experience

Assisted living facilities are a model of care provision which is increasingly used by relatively wealthy older persons to build a bridge between living independently at one's own home and living in a residential or long-term care facility. There are, however, important differences across countries in the degree of public financing available for receiving care services in such a setting as well as in government involvement to overview quality of services delivered. Considerable private saving or insurance coverage is often required to make this care choice financially feasible for the individual.

The so-called "group-living" initiative for dementia patients is an example of ways in which the long-term care market has evolved to reflect preferences of patients and their families (Moïse et al., 2004). Across the OECD, nursing homes are increasingly setting aside units focused exclusively on care for dementia patients. The idea is to allow staff to better handle difficult behavioural problems, thus achieving better care for dementia patients without compromising care of other residents. Group-living exists in significant numbers in OECD countries such as France, Japan, Spain, Sweden, and the United States and is becoming increasingly popular. However, as is the case with so many organisational innovations in health care, evidence on the relative benefits and costs of group-living is lacking (Doody et al., 2001).

Greater control by individual consumers over long-term care spending

A number of countries have reformed their policies to allow more consumer choice. Two approaches that have been adopted are:

- Personal budgets and consumer-directed employment of care assistants (*e.g.* Netherlands, Norway, some US states; direct payments are being expanded in the United Kingdom).

- Payment to the person needing care to spend as they wish to achieve sufficient care (*e.g.* Austria, France, Germany).

As rated by the older person needing care and their main care-giver, the experience with these initiatives has been positive, reflecting increased flexibility and control over services received, and reduced feelings of dependency (Lundsgaard, 2004).

Unless limited by a cap on budget or benefits, consumer-directed spending policies are likely to be more expensive than traditional approaches for covering services. While experience suggests that consumer-directed spending will not necessarily be a low-cost option, there are also grounds for suggesting it does not necessarily have to be more costly. Most people, given the choice, will choose to remain in their own home to receive care. A number of studies have shown that there are many disabled older people, particularly those who have support from an informal caregiver, for whom the home-based option can be less expensive than entry to an institution.[4] Additionally, in Germany, where since 1996 disabled older people have been given a choice of receiving either a package of services or a (less costly) care allowance, two-thirds of beneficiaries have opted for the lower-cost care allowance to spend as they wish. Independence has a value to older people that can outweigh the offer of more expensive forms of care.

Health insurance options can increase the responsiveness of health systems

One of the main policy goals in many of the OECD health systems that have a role for private health insurance is increased consumer satisfaction and increased responsiveness of health systems to consumer preferences. By offering an array of differentiated products, private health insurance markets can increase consumers' choice of benefits and financial protection schemes – especially when choice is accompanied by accessible and usable information to compare options. Those who choose to purchase private health insurance often have a greater array of providers, treatments, or options in terms of timeliness of care from which to choose. In addition, and perhaps more importantly, health systems as a whole may become more responsive to consumer preferences to the extent that persons are able to select and to change their health coverage and providers.

The availability of private health insurance enhances consumer choice in many of the countries where it serves as optional duplicate coverage for patients eligible for publicly financed care. In Australia, for example, patients who have private insurance can use private hospitals and choose their own doctors in both public and private hospitals. And in Ireland, those with private insurance have access to private hospitals that are not reimbursed under the public system. In the US Medicare program, most beneficiaries have the option to enrol in a privately administered health insurance plan that usually offers less choice of provider but more benefits and lower cost-sharing.[5]

The availability of private supplemental insurance policies enhances choice of covered benefits, as does complementary insurance with respect to cost-sharing arrangements and the degree of risk pooling. For example, US Medicare beneficiaries have a choice of up to ten different packages designed to cover patient cost-sharing and offer different benefits not covered in the publicly financed programme.[6] A small market of supplemental long-term care insurance is developing in a few OECD countries where public programmes of coverage have expanded (e.g. France, Germany), reflecting differences in consumers' willingness to risk the large cost-sharing requirements associated with these schemes.

The greatest scope for improved choice and responsiveness arguably occurs where there are multiple insurers that serve as the primary source of coverage for some portions of the population. This depends greatly on the regulatory requirements established to set ground rules, however. For example, in many markets in the United States, there is significant variation across private insurance products in size and inclusiveness of provider network, benefits covered, cost-sharing arrangements, the financial incentives under which providers operate, and demand management rules. Limited regulatory constraints on insurance arrangements, combined with a relatively high level of choice,[7] can encourage innovation in approaches to health-care financing and delivery. Reflecting these factors, US markets are quick to respond to purchaser (individual and employer) preferences (Docteur et al., 2003).[8] In Switzerland, on the other hand, there is much less variation in both mandatory health insurance and supplementary insurance products, partly due to regulation designed to ensure equity of access and financing. Here, health insurance products differ primarily in terms of premium cost.

Lack of accessible information limits the ability of insured persons to take meaningful advantage of choice in private health insurance products, as it is often difficult to compare insurer offerings by price and benefits. This is one plausible explanation for limited consumer switching of insurers for basic, compulsory social insurance coverage in Switzerland (Colombo, 2001). Information deficiencies have also been found to be an issue in social health insurance systems that have attempted to introduce competition across social insurers, as in the Netherlands and Germany (Gress et al., 2002). Australia and some US states[9] have developed comparative information for consumers to use in making choices and have provided guidelines for industry-produced information.

Permitting insurers to differentiate their products through benefits and provider differences is necessary to reveal consumer preferences. However, extensive product differentiation carries risk of increasing consumer confusion and undermining risk pooling in insurance markets. Disclosure requirements can be used to promote consumers' understanding of their complex product options and help promote meaningful choice within the private health insurance market. Steps to promote availability and affordability of insurance for high-risk persons (such as those described in Box 2.2) may be needed if policy makers are concerned about differences in equity that can arise.

Approaches for increasing system responsiveness: summary of findings

Moderate waiting times do not appear to have negative effects on health outcomes, but they do affect quality of life and are likely to entail some costs borne outside the health system, such as in terms of worker productivity. Countries will weight these costs differently when deciding whether or what action to redress waiting times problems is appropriate. Countries' decisions may vary also, depending on how they view equity considerations with respect to elective care, and whether they believe that it is appropriate to ration certain services according to willingness to pay. Those countries that wish to reduce waiting times judged to be excessive will need to either increase surgical capacity or increase productivity, recognising that the former will result in cost increases, as may the latter. However, if the supply of surgery is judged to be adequate, waiting times can be reduced by changing the propensity to generate waiting through, for example, management of demand or provision of financial incentives for doctors to reduce lists.

The question of how private health insurance can be employed so as to increase health-system responsiveness is a difficult one.[10] The availability of coverage options in and of itself creates more consumer choice, although the extent to which that choice is meaningful depends largely on the extent of variation across products. It is clear that a system of multiple private or social insurers that are free to innovate is likely to evolve in line with consumer preferences in a way that is difficult for single-payer systems to do. But the financial cost (assessed later in this report) and cost to equity can be considerable, and difficult to overcome.

Notes

1. Because most patients lack the information needed to evaluate the quality of care furnished on the basis of their experiences, patient satisfaction may be more highly influenced by other factors. Efforts by policy makers and other stakeholders to increase the availability and usability of information on technical quality of care and other aspects of performance that benefit from more informed or systematic assessment may change matters in the future.

2. For example, take-up of duplicate private health insurance is less than 15% in Portugal, Spain, and the United Kingdom, even though speedier access to care is a main motivation for private insurance purchase in these countries.

3. For example, Propper (1990 and 1995) found that respondents in England were willing to pay only around USD 100 in 2001 prices to reduce waiting for surgery for stable elective conditions by one month. Bishai and Lang (2000) came up with a range of estimates of willingness to pay for reducing waiting for cataract surgery of between USD 30 and USD 130 per month in Canada, Denmark and Spain.

4. See, for example, for the United Kingdom, Tinker et al. (1999).

5. Because such insurance is paid mostly through public financing (Medicare beneficiaries generally pay only a small premium), this coverage is technically not considered private health insurance by the OECD's definition.

6. Not all packages are available for sale in all markets, partly reflecting premium escalation caused by adverse selection against plans that offer the most comprehensive benefits.

7. The extent of choice varies. Many employers offer more than one insurance plan from which employees can choose, although some offer only one or none. Those purchasing products on the individual market may have less choice or even no access to coverage, particularly if they fall into higher-risk groups.

8. This is evidenced, for example, by the quick changes in coverage arrangements following the so-called backlash against managed care, which resulted in a proliferation of more loosely managed insurance products.

9. The federal government and the states also jointly prepare and distribute comparative coverage information on Medicare supplemental insurance policies.

10. In making policy decisions as to the appropriate role of private health insurance in a health system, it is important to recognise that many, if not most of the policy-relevant characteristics are design characteristics, rather than intrinsic ones. Whether such coverage is voluntary or mandatory; whether coverage substitutes for, duplicates, supplements or complements public coverage; whether insurers compete and on what grounds; and what government interventions (e.g. market regulations, subsidies) are employed are all critical factors in determining the impact of private health insurance on a health system.

ISBN 92-64-01555-8
Towards High-Performing Health Systems
© OECD 2004

Chapter 4

Health-care spending: the quest for affordable costs and sustainable financing

Rising health costs continue to be a pressing policy issue in most OECD countries, although the nature of the concerns has changed somewhat over time. Most OECD countries have employed, with some success, tools to contain the rate of increase in spending. However, these initiatives invariably failed to address the root causes of spending growth and, in some cases, had unwanted side-effects, such as creation or exacerbation of waiting times for certain services. Furthermore, some countries have found their cost-containment efforts to be too successful and are now considering whether systems are funded adequately to meet performance objectives.

Rising costs and their impact

Rising health costs

Health represents an important share of OECD member country economies, constituting more than 8% of GDP, on average, and more than 10% of the economy in three OECD countries in 2001 (Figure 4.1). Health-care costs have risen steadily over the past decade in all

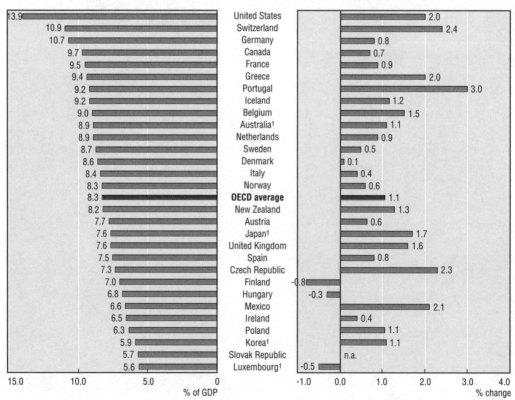

Figure 4.1. **Health expenditure as a percentage of GDP, 2001**

Figure 4.2. **Change in total health expenditure as a percentage of GDP, 1990-2001**

Note: The average change in total health expenditure excludes the Slovak Republic and Turkey. It includes 2000 data, in place of 2001 data, for Australia, Japan, Korea and Luxembourg and 1992 data, in place of 1990 data, for Germany.
1. 2000.

Source: OECD Health Data 2003.

Figure 4.3. **Share of the population aged 80 and over, 2000**

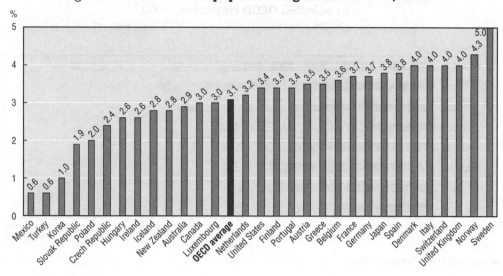

Source: OECD Health Data 2003.

OECD countries and, in most countries, health expenditure increased at a faster rate than their economies as a whole (Figure 4.2).

Advances in the capability of medicine to treat and prevent health conditions are widely agreed to be a major factor driving health cost growth, responsible for as much as half of total increases in costs over the past half-century (Newhouse, 1992). New technologies – the conquest of infectious diseases by new vaccines, the development of therapies for many previously untreatable conditions such as AIDS, and now the emergence of genome-based approaches – transformed the practice of medicine during this period. Recent developments in imaging, biotechnology, and pharmacology suggest that this trend is likely to continue (Aaron, 2003).

The implications of population ageing for health-care costs are an important consideration. OECD populations are ageing rapidly. Across OECD countries, life expectancy has grown over the past four decades at an average rate of 2.3 months each year, and a low birth rate means that younger cohorts are falling in size. These two tendencies mean that, in particular, the share of the population aged 80 and over now exceeds 3% and is growing in most OECD countries (Figure 4.3).

It is not clear whether population ageing itself will place greater strains on the acute-care system. There is evidence that care costs for any individual are concentrated in the last two years of life, and that the total cost of care for the elderly is the same for different life expectancies. If this continues to be the case as populations age, care costs also will be deferred. On the other hand, the number of older people in the population is certain to increase rapidly and, as these people have a higher mortality rate, the share of individuals in their last years of life will increase. OECD projections based on average public spending by age group[1] suggest that health costs will increase by approximately 2 percentage points of GDP over the period 2000-2050 (Bains and Oxley, 2004). As this does not take into account the effects of delayed mortality, it probably represents an upward bound of the impact of ageing.

Rising long-term care costs

Public and private expenditures on long-term care services for older persons are rising in OECD countries. There has been strong growth in the number of very elderly people, the age group

Figure 4.4. **Public expenditure on long-term care as a share of GDP in selected OECD countries, 2000**

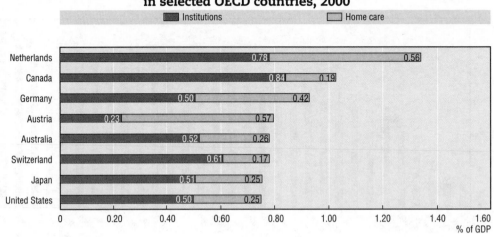

Source: OECD Long-Term Care Study.

in which need for long-term care is most pronounced. In many countries (*e.g.* Australia, Germany, Japan and Luxembourg), recent public expenditure growth has been driven by expansions of public programmes to assist dependent persons in need of care. More generally, expenditures on long-term care are rising in many countries in response to growing expectations of an ageing population, changes in family structure and living conditions of older persons (OECD, 2004b).[2]

Long-term care costs currently represent a relatively small proportion of GDP, by comparison with health,[3] in part reflecting the prevalence of unpaid caregiving at home (Figure 4.4). However, the high projected growth rate of older age groups means that public spending on long-term care services is likely to at least double, on average, as a share of GDP by 2050, according to OECD projections (Bains and Oxley, 2004). This increase could be higher if other factors, such as higher unit-cost increases or reduced family care, create higher demand than currently from these age groups. This projected increase could also be lower if very elderly people in the future enjoy better health and lower levels of disability. Given the uncertainty about trends in these factors, it is important for policies to be sufficiently flexible to adapt to future circumstances.

Costs put pressure on public budgets

In most OECD countries, concern about continued growth in health costs reflects the pressure such growth places on public budgets. Given the predominance of publicly financed coverage or direct public financing of care in most OECD countries, the public sector accounts for the greatest part of health spending (72% on average) in all countries except Korea, Mexico, and the United States (Figure 4.5). And even in the United States, where the private sector plays an unusually large role in financing, public expenditure on health represents 6% of GDP, comparable to the OECD average percentage represented by public spending (OECD, 2003d).

There are wide differences across countries in the share of long-term care spending borne publicly (*e.g.* about 60% in the United States, more than 90% in the Netherlands) (Figure 4.6). Several countries have increased spending on home care services, but not all of these countries are similarly increasing the resources spent on care provided in institutions. Where new public programs have eased access to both home care and institutional care, both components may in fact be on the rise, as, for example, has occurred in Germany over the past ten years (OECD, 2004b).

Figure 4.5. **Per capita expenditure on health, 2001**

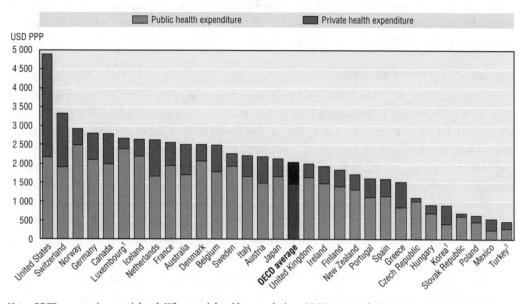

Note: OECD average is unweighted. When weighted by population, OECD average is USD 2 535 PPP per capita.
1. 2000.
Source: OECD Health Data 2003; data for Turkey are from Turkish National Health Accounts.

Figure 4.6. **Long-term care expenditure by source of financing in selected OECD countries, 2000**

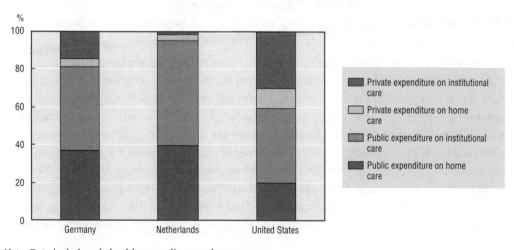

Note: Data include only health expenditure on long term care.
Source: OECD Long-Term Care Study.

The experience with health-care cost containment

Although countries have had some short-term success in containing costs, coping with cost pressure continues to be a pressing problem in many OECD countries.

Approaches used in cost-containment efforts

Faced with a rising trend in health spending, most OECD countries have sought to rein in this growth over the past two decades. Typically, the approaches used to slow the growth in spending have relied on cost-containment policies, such as i) regulation of prices, input resources and (to a lesser extent) health-care service volumes; ii) caps on health spending, either overall or by sector; and iii) shifts of costs onto private sources of financing (individual patients or private health insurance).

Regulation of prices and supply

Most countries regulate health-sector prices and/or service volumes in some fashion, often in ways intended to influence both public and private spending levels. Wage controls are prevalent in systems where most of the health-care workers are public-sector employees, as they are in the Nordic countries, Greece, Italy, and Portugal. In other systems, payments for medical services, supplies, and institutional care are usually set administratively, or governments provide oversight on prices agreed between health-care purchasers and providers. In the United Kingdom, the government regulates the domestic profits of pharmaceutical companies. Most countries take steps to influence service volumes, ranging from controls over medical school admissions and other workforce policies to more direct efforts to control hospital sector capacity.

The impact of price controls on health expenditure can be limited by provider responses in some cases, as experience has shown that health-care providers respond to the economic incentives established in payment systems. For example, to compensate for price limits, practitioners may increase the volume of services provided or change the mix of services to include more of those paid at a higher rate,[4] as occurred in Korea until fees were increased in the mid-1990s (OECD, 2003e). Sometimes services are shifted into sectors or systems where there are no price controls, something that has occurred in some countries where public and private programs operate side-by-side, as in Greece and Ireland.[5] And patients may be up-coded to higher level payment classifications, where such differentiation is built into payment systems.

Other factors influencing the success of price controls as a cost-containment tool include the administrative costs associated with their use and whether prices are set at levels that correspond to the costs of health-care delivery by an efficient provider. A more important limitation over the longer term is that long periods of wage or price restraint can seriously limit the ability of the health-care sector to attract qualified personnel and maintain health-care capacity. Nevertheless, sophisticated payment systems have been used successfully, where they are accompanied by careful monitoring of impact. Notably, the US Medicare programme has implemented complex prospective payment systems for most types of health-care services that are credited with slowing the rate of cost growth as well as improving the cost-effectiveness of health-care delivery. These systems have been adopted for use by private payers.

Caps on health spending

Budgetary caps or controls have been widely used as an instrument for containing expenditure. Initially, these were directed at the hospital sector, the most costly element of the system. They were subsequently extended to other providers and suppliers so as to improve ability to control overall expenditure, particularly given the potential for substitution across sectors. Spending controls now often include global budgets spanning all components of public spending on health and supplementary spending caps on ambulatory care and pharmaceuticals.

In general, use of budgetary caps to control spending appears to have been most successful in countries where health-care delivery is a public-sector responsibility – as in Denmark, Ireland, and New Zealand – and in single-payer countries, like Canada. Where budget limits are firm and enforceable, they can serve as a powerful tool to limit spending. However, top-down spending constraints in the form of budget caps can also have undesirable incentive effects in that they can provide little incentive for providers to make efficiency gains or increase productivity. For example, fixed budget ceilings encourage providers and suppliers to spend up to the ceiling. Setting budgets based on historical costs may favour inefficient providers and penalize efficient ones. As a consequence, OECD countries have been moving increasingly to combine budget caps with measures that take account of levels of output and relative efficiency across hospitals.

Shifting spending to the private sector

Some OECD countries have taken steps to reduce the burden of health costs on public financing systems. Patterns are different across the OECD. In some countries, patient cost sharing has increased as a result of policy changes. And in some of these countries, this has been accompanied by growth in private health insurance. Although in some cases these efforts have succeeded in reducing the public finance burden, the impact of such initiatives on total spending has been minimal.

Impact of cost-sharing increases on public and total spending. Cost-sharing measures appear to have had an impact on the share of public spending in total spending. Following large increases relating to the expansion of publicly financed coverage schemes for health-care services in the 1970s, the increase in the public share of total health spending slowed markedly in the 1980s. Between 1990 and 2000, the average share of total health spending represented by the public sector was stable at about 72%.[6]

The impact of cost-shifting policies on overall household demand and consumption of health-care has been limited, however, given that cost-sharing requirements remain minimal in most OECD countries and where they are larger, protections for high-cost users and low-income persons are generally used. Available empirical evidence suggests that the elasticity of demand for health care is generally small, with the weakest response at the level of hospital care.[7] Nevertheless, large co-payments can have a real impact on demand for services (see Box 4.1).

Role of private health insurance in public and total cost containment. Some countries have promoted the development of private health insurance markets as a means to reduce demand and cost pressures on public health systems. They have done so by allowing private insurance to duplicate the coverage provided in the public programme (e.g. Australia, Ireland, United Kingdom), by having entire groups within the population rely on private, rather than public coverage (e.g. Germany, Netherlands, United States), or by excluding services from public coverage (e.g. dental care in the Netherlands).

While private health insurance accounts for an average of only 6.4% of total health expenditure in OECD countries and only 23% of all private health expenditure, there is great heterogeneity across countries.[8] Few countries have seen notable changes in the share of total health expenditure covered by private health insurance over the past decade,[9] although some countries have seen expansions in the share of population covered (OECD, 2004c).

> ### Box 4.1. **Effect of cost-sharing on health cost containment in Korea**
>
> In Korea, out-of-pocket payments represent 41% of total health expenditure, the second-highest share in OECD countries (OECD, 2003c). This is due to large co-payments and exclusion of certain types of services from coverage by the National Health Insurance (NHI) system. Coverage exclusions and high out-of-pocket costs are among the likely factors explaining why Korea's per capita health expenditure lies below what could be expected for a country with its standard of living.
>
> Large co-payments have not been sufficient to contain growth in health spending nor to maintain fiscal balance within the NHI system, however. In fact, the annual rate of growth in real per capita health expenditure has since 1985 remained well above the annual growth of real GDP per capita, with the exception of a few years. The trend for public spending alone has been similar. The financial position of the NHI has been deteriorating since the beginning of the 1990s, mainly led by growth in volumes of health services. Structural factors, such as population ageing and rising expectations by the population for more and better care, as well as the incentives created by fee-for-service reimbursement within a profit-oriented environment, are behind such growth. The NHI system started to operate in deficit since 1995. After the introduction of two major reforms in 2000, expenditure in the NHI system skyrocketed, turning pre-existing deficits into a dramatic financial crisis.
>
> *Source:* OECD (2003e).

Private insurance that duplicates public coverage has taken on some costs that would otherwise have been borne publicly. For example, private health insurance has helped to finance increases in private hospital capacity in Australia and may have helped to relieve financial pressures on public hospitals that also treat privately insured patients, as in Australia and Ireland. However, the extent to which health costs have been shifted to private insurance has been limited. Often, private health insurers concentrate on treating minor risks, while the cost of more costly cases and services rest with the public system, as in the United Kingdom and Ireland.[10] In Australia, many privately insured patients continue to use publicly financed health-care services. In the United States, Medicare beneficiaries who have chosen to enrol in privately administered insurance plans can disenrol and return to the traditional, publicly administered programme when they have serious illnesses so as to increase their choice of providers and treatments.[11] This benefits the private insurers at the expense of public financing.

Although public spending may be lower than it would otherwise be in countries that restrict access to public coverage for certain population groups, it is notable that public spending represents a relatively high share of GDP in those countries. This may be largely explained by the fact that private markets tend to cover relatively healthier and lower-risk persons, while higher risks and/or older cohorts, representing the large majority of total health spending, are enrolled in public programmes. Similarly, excluding services from coverage surely relieves public systems of some costs, but the type of services that are excluded (*e.g.* optical and dental care) do not normally represent a significant source of costs. The extent to which such costs are picked up by private insurers, as opposed to out-of-pocket spending by patients, varies across countries.

There is also the risk that private health insurance can have an *increasing* effect on public expenditure. For example, private health insurance coverage of co-payments on publicly financed health services, as in France, erodes price signals and incentives for patients to consume care parsimoniously, tending to increase demand for services. Coverage may be important to ensure access, however, where patient cost sharing is relatively high, as in the US Medicare programme. Also, private health insurance may increase burdens on the public sector if the cost of any subsidy directed to private cover more than compensates for savings derived from cost shifting. Furthermore, particularly where supply is tight, private insurers may bid up prices paid by public payers.

Countries that have multiple sources of primary insurance coverage (private and social) are among the ones with the highest total health expenditure,[12] suggesting that such institutional arrangements are more costly. Cost control is more problematic to achieve in multiple-payer systems because the purchasers have less power in bargaining with providers over prices and quantities, unless universal reimbursement limits or cost controls are established, as they are in Switzerland. Absent public intervention, the prices paid by private insurers are likely to be higher than the administered prices set or negotiated by public payers, as private insurers in most countries do not have extensive market share (although here Ireland serves as an exception). Countries tend to apply cost-containment measures to the public system only, although there are exceptions, as in the Netherlands. In addition, systems based on private health insurance also tend to have higher administrative costs, as compared with single-payer social insurance[13] or public-integrated systems.[14] This may reflect higher costs incurred by insurers in a competitive environment.[15] Dealing with multiple insurers may also increase the administrative costs of providers.

If private health insurance is to be used to reduce the public financing burden, a number of practices may be usefully employed (OECD, 2004c). First, in systems where private coverage duplicates public, policies should encourage privately insured patients to use privately financed care, recognising that private insurance premiums will rise accordingly. Second, public financing savings arising from a transfer of health costs to private health insurance need to be weighted against the cost of any subsidy towards private insurance markets. Third, prohibiting private health insurance coverage of modest co-payments may be helpful to counteract moral hazard, although some form of such coverage may be needed to safeguard access for vulnerable populations or for others where co-payments are large. Fourth, policy-makers should consider applying cost-containment measures (such as administered-pricing schemes) to both public and private financing to have the greatest impact on both public and total spending.

Success in containing the rate of health-cost growth

Cost-containment efforts such as those described above coincided with a decline in the rate of spending growth across many OECD countries. On average, the annual growth rate in real health expenditures during the 1980s (3.2%) and 1990s (3.0%), when many cost-containment initiatives were undertaken, was considerably slower than it was in the 1970s (6.0%). Despite some apparent short-run success in slowing the rate of health cost increases, however, cost-containment measures have generally not addressed the underlying source of cost growth pressures, and health cost increases (total and public, in most cases) still exceeded average economic growth in most OECD countries during the 1990s. Spending has picked up again in the early part of this decade.

Judging the appropriateness of health spending levels

A rising health spending to GDP ratio is not necessarily problematic from a policy perspective. Indeed, social welfare may well be improved by increased spending, particularly if demand for health-care services tends to rise more rapidly than income and if the cost of technological change is more than compensated by improvements in the quality of care and resulting health outcomes.

Adding to this is the fact that the trade-offs and consequences (intended and unintended) of cost-containment initiatives are well-recognized. For example, capped budgets create incentives to adopt cost-saving technologies, but create disincentives to take up technologies that may be cost-effective but cost-increasing, or that may reduce costs on a per-unit base but drive up overall costs because of resulting growth in volume. Similarly, administered pricing systems may not result in payment levels that reflect the value of the product and the cost of production, resulting in market distortions. For example, Halm and Gelijns (1991) cite an example of administered prices for cochlear implants in the US Medicare program being set at a level that covered only a fraction of the cost of the device. This led to under-diffusion and had a negative impact on subsequent investment in research and development.

Nevertheless, policy makers must make decisions regarding the value of spending in the health sector versus competing priorities for scarce resources. Indeed, an emerging dilemma facing governments is judging the "appropriate" level of health spending.

In general, OECD countries with higher per capita GDP tend to spend more per capita on health (Figure 4.7). The effect of income on health spending appears to reflect income's impact on both volume and price of services, in that both the amount of health-care consumption and the relatively labour-intensive prices of health services tend to be greater at higher income levels. There is significant variation across countries, however, which may partly reflect policy decisions regarding appropriate spending levels and the perceived value of additional spending on health relative to other goods and services. This variation, combined with evidence that the income-spending relationship is weaker for the richest OECD countries, further suggests that income growth need not necessarily result in increased health spending. Rather, policy decisions and design characteristics of systems can play a significant role in determining the extent of income-driven growth.

In considering the appropriate response to pressures for increased spending, it is worth noting that the level of resources required to reach performance goals will vary, depending on the level of performance sought and the inputs required for a particular set of institutional arrangements.[16] Comparative data on system characteristics, inputs, and outputs across countries can be of significant value in making such assessments. For example, OECD work has documented a relationship between health-spending levels and waiting times for elective surgery (Siciliani and Hurst, 2003). An increase in public expenditure per capita of USD 100 was associated with a reduction of 5.6 days in the mean waiting time across countries, while an increase of USD 100 per capita in total spending was associated with a reduction in waiting times of 6.6 days. However, decisions to increase spending on health may not necessarily have the desired impact on performance and countries will value potential improvements differently (see Box 4.2). In addition, considerations of what is affordable, given financing capacity, will also vary across countries.

Figure 4.7. **Health expenditure and GDP per capita, 2001**

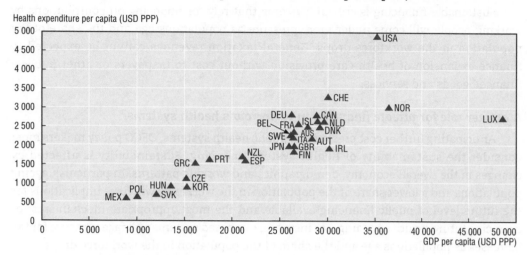

Source: OECD Health Data 2003.

Box 4.2. **Are waiting times indicative of shortfalls in public spending on health care?**

Numerous factors put upward pressure on the volume of elective surgery in OECD countries. If surgery is provided free, or almost free, of charge, as it is in many OECD health systems, the cost sensitivity of prospective patients will be low. Also, demand for elective interventions may be "induced" by surgeons when they, or the units in which they work, are paid on a fee-for-service or activity-related basis, respectively. Across and within countries, surgeons disagree on the indications for much elective surgery.

However, policy makers must consider costs as well as benefits, and, ultimately, the fiscal capacity to finance public programmes. They will generally be unwilling to allow public services to be "demand led" either by patients or by doctors. That leads them, in some cases, to impose budget limits and capacity constraints on surgery. It may also lead them to avoid activity-related payment mechanisms in the interests of cost containment. Further, it may lead them to take steps to manage demand. The (implicit) aim will be to set surgery rates at the socially desirable level which balances marginal benefits with marginal costs. Such "non-price" rationing may result in waiting lists. In effect, waiting times for elective surgery take the place of prices in controlling demand.

There is room for much variation in judgements in setting budgets and capacity for surgery. If surgeons are uncertain about indications for, and effectiveness of, elective surgery, policy makers cannot be expected to find it easy to make judgements about budgets and capacity. Ultimately, much will depend on the relative value assigned to system responsiveness and timeliness of improvements in the quality of life of prospective patients compared with the costs incurred by increasing capacity and activity, or by taking other steps to reduce waiting. The final judgement will always rest with governments (and their electorate) where publicly funded surgery is concerned.

Sustainable financing for health and long-term care

Sustainable financing is critical. Systems that rely for financing on contributions by working people will come under more pressure as populations age and the share of the population in the workforce drops. General taxation revenues cannot be expected to finance expansion of health-care provision without cost to taxpayers or other publicly financed goods and services.

A greater role for private financing in tomorrow's health systems?

Anticipating further cost pressure on public health systems, OECD policy makers must consider the sustainability of health-system financing. Sustainability is affected by changes in the overall economy, demographics and working patterns. In particular, ageing populations and a lower share of the population in the workforce will have implications for the future level of public financing available and the most appropriate mechanisms for financing future health spending. For instance, tax-based systems will face pressure for tax increases as populations age and the share of the population in the workforce drops.

Changes of this type are likely to bring to the forefront questions about the appropriate role for private financing of health systems. Increasing user fees is one approach, although the impact of modest cost-sharing on total spending is relatively low, particularly if exemptions and caps are used or if private health insurance covers the user fees. Delisting services that are considered of low benefit may be worthwhile where public coverage is generous, although the total impact on public financing may not be great. Eligibility for publicly financed cover could be reduced, although this risks solidarity. Policy makers may wish to employ private health insurance that duplicates public coverage to increase total financing where public resources or supply of publicly financed providers is judged inadequate. However, experience has shown that using private insurance in this manner is challenging for a number of reasons. First, people must be motivated to buy private insurance, meaning that they perceive that public coverage fails to meet their needs. Then, they must be motivated to use privately financed services. Some OECD countries have used subsidies and regulation so as to obtain the desired ends, but it is not clear that these have been achieved.

Increasing the private share of health financing also raises issues as to financing equity. Because private health insurance premiums are generally not income-based, and often vary by age, as well as health status factors – at least to some degree, private health insurance tends to be a more regressive source of financing than most public or social insurance systems. It is, however, more progressive than out-of-pocket payments, in that it provides individuals with a means of pooling health-care costs. Government efforts to promote access to private health insurance through restrictions on risk selection or targeted subsidies can improve the equity of private health insurance markets in terms of financing, although this carries costs (see Box 2.2 above).

Financing long-term care services: individual or collective approaches?

Financing the care that elderly people need to remain functional has become a fraught issue in many countries, given shifts in population composition and changes in financing capacity. Incomes of older generations have risen compared with those at the start of their careers (OECD, 2001). Furthermore, the ratio of working population to elderly is declining across the OECD (Dang et al., 2001). These developments imply that financing changes that take into account such changes in ability to pay may be appropriate. For example, the income of elderly people themselves may be needed to meet some of the burden, or other means, such as the introduction of a new pillar in welfare systems, will have to be found.

Recent financing changes in a number of OECD countries have reflected these developments. A number of countries (*e.g.* Germany, Japan, Luxembourg) have implemented social insurance coverage for long-term care and a number of other countries (*e.g.* France, Korea) are considering doing so (see Box 4.3). Relatively few countries – among them Australia and the Netherlands – have for some time provided long-term care coverage within their public systems of financing for health care. Some countries in which long-term care services have been provided on relatively generous terms have acted to improve future sustainability by increasing the share of the cost borne by clients who can afford it (*e.g.* Australia, Sweden, some Canadian provinces).

Private long-term care insurance does not currently play a significant role in funding long-term care services (see Box 4.4). A special type of private insurance arrangement has been created in Germany with the introduction of social long-term care insurance, where the additional coverage of long-term care risks for 8% of the population became mandatory for private health insurance companies under rules of eligibility and risk-sharing that closely resemble those of the social insurance system. Complementary long-term care insurance on top of public coverage is a growing market in several countries, but these contracts are typically marketed to consumers who will not become recipients in the near future, and so do not result in much current expenditure on services (other than on insurance administration).

It is also noteworthy that, while delivery of long-term care is frequently a regional or local policy issue, in some countries, decisions regarding the financial terms for users also rest with sub-national governments (*e.g.* Canada, Spain and Switzerland). Having different terms applicable dependent on where one lives has led to debates about whether long-term care should have a similar degree of national guidance as acute health care in these countries.

Equity considerations in long-term care financing

One major debate around equity in long-term care has focused on how the cost of care can most reasonably be shared between individuals, and whatever forms of collective risk sharing could be employed. The cost of long-term care is a significant risk that falls to some older people and their families and not to others. While many older people may require some help at home, the most catastrophic costs of nursing home care, or its equivalent delivered in one's own home, cannot be met by many older people without draining their personal resources. In addition, insuring against these risks remains very expensive when undertaken on an individual basis because those with greater likelihood of need are more likely to seek insurance. If purchase of such insurance were mandatory, premiums would benefit from the risk pooling.

For these reasons, a growing number of countries have chosen a form of collective social insurance to help meet the most severe costs of long-term care, in the same way that societies provide collective insurance against the risk of illness and of disability at a young age. There are, however, differences evident in the degree to which countries aim to achieve equity of access to long-term care independent of ability to pay. Besides social insurance solutions, other countries have defined the public responsibility for long-term care to be more one of a safety-net for cases where private means are inadequate.

Box 4.3. **Social long-term care insurance for ageing societies: recent experience in Germany and Japan**

Many OECD countries use mandatory social insurance to fund social programmes such as retirement pensions, disability pensions and health care. Facing a rising demand for long-term care in an ageing society, a number of countries have been considering this means of covering the associated rising costs to society. Both Germany and Japan have mandatory social insurance for other risks and have extended their range of social insurance schemes to cover long-term care, in 1995/1996 and 2000 respectively.

In both countries rising costs of long-term care were falling on other public budgets which were neither adequate nor designed to cover this. In Germany during the late 1980s and early 1990s the number of elderly people receiving means-tested social assistance went up significantly, as increasing numbers could not meet the cost of long-term care, mainly in institutions, and had to rely on social assistance after spending down their savings. An addition to the compulsory social insurance scheme addressed these problems for most long-term care users and provided a boost towards home care in preference to institutional care.

In Japan, public expenditure on long-term care increased in the 1980s and 1990s, through the increase of long-term care in tax-funded social services and the inappropriate use of hospital care funded by health insurance. It was seen as necessary to raise a new source of finance for long-term care and to re-draw the boundaries of the existing health insurance to focus on acute care.

In both countries the new long-term care insurance was well received by the public, although additional contributions were required from both working age and retired people (age 40 and older in Japan). There were a number of similar factors contributing to success: Both countries had a long tradition of covering major social and health risks through mandatory social insurance, and previous experience of administering public health insurance aided the implementation process as government could call upon a framework of existing social protection mechanisms (health insurance bodies in Germany and municipalities in Japan). In both countries there was a strong public concern about the need for long-term care in old age and therefore an acceptance of the additional contributions.

Common policy challenges remain. In both countries the new schemes succeeded in alleviating pressure on other public budgets, and in supporting the growth of new long-term care providers, including a broader range of home care services. However, the rising numbers of older people together with low macroeconomic performance have recently put these systems under some strain. In Germany, the contribution rate is fixed by law at 1.7% of pay (up to a ceiling), and the scheme has seen growing deficits in 2002 and 2003. However, benefit rates are not index-linked and have not been increased. In Japan, three years after introduction most municipalities had to increase insurance premiums by around 10%. Although the Japanese government is promoting effective use of services by adjusting the rate of remuneration, and closer inspection of expenses incurred, a further increase in premiums appears inevitable.

Box 4.4. **Private long-term care insurance: experience and challenges**

The very high cost of formal long-term care and the concentration of need for care among the elderly suggest that long-term care services may be most appropriately financed through a collective risk-pooling mechanism. Some have argued that public programmes may best perform this function, and indeed, policy makers in several countries have made this decision. However, in other cases countries have decided to place the long-term care financing burden somewhat or primarily on private financing. The question then arises as to whether private insurance mechanisms provide a useful way to spread the risk of these costs across the population, and which populations (by age, risk or income categories) can most benefit from these pooling efforts.

There is little experience with private long-term care insurance in OECD countries to draw upon in considering these issues. Despite a growing role in a limited number of countries (*e.g.* France and the United States), voluntary private long-term care insurance is currently not a major source of financing long-term care in any OECD member country. It plays the largest role in the United States, where private insurance represents 11% of total spending on long-term care.

Challenges confronting private long-term care insurance markets – and possible reasons for limited development – include low levels of purchase by non-elderly, poor consumer retention of policies, difficulties projecting future costs and incidence, premium stability, and the advantages and disadvantages of purchasing insurance versus self-funding at different income levels.

Approaches for pursuing affordable costs and sustainable financing: summary of findings

Methods and means for controlling the rate of public spending growth are now widely available in most OECD countries, using a combination of budgetary and administrative controls over payments, prices, and supply of services. Although sophisticated administered-pricing systems can be technically difficult to employ, there are numerous examples of successful systems that promote productivity without evident harm to outcomes. Over the long term, keeping wages and prices at unrealistically low levels is likely to have a distorting and undesirable effect on markets, so vigilance is required.

Establishing modest cost-sharing requirements may be appropriate when policy makers wish to reduce the burden on public systems of financing. Nevertheless, policy-makers should not expect big savings from this approach, particularly as vulnerable populations must be exempted to avoid restrictions on access that could be costly in the long run. This will impose administrative costs. And reduced demand for health services will not necessarily enhance efficiency, given that consumers are equally likely to skimp on preventive care and appropriate treatments unless given incentives to do otherwise. Also, allowing private health insurance to cover modest cost-sharing amounts eliminates the demand-reducing effect of cost sharing and might have cost-increasing effects, in aggregate.

In any case, advances in health care and the increased demand inherent in increasingly wealthy and ageing populations mean that continued cost pressure is virtually inevitable. Countries must choose the appropriate response and find health spending levels that are suitable to needs and circumstances, given a particular set of institutional characteristics, performance objectives, affordability considerations, and the sustainability of financing. The ageing of OECD populations, the higher incomes of older persons, expectations for economic growth, and equity considerations must all be taken into account. While richer countries tend to spend more on health, there is great variation in spending among countries with comparable incomes, and great room for policy decision making to impact spending levels.

There is a strong case for ensuring that people are protected against the risk of incurring catastrophic expenses for long-term care, as is the norm in the areas of acute health-care and disability. This can be achieved through different approaches, such as mandatory public insurance (Luxembourg, Netherlands and Japan), a mix of public and mandatory private insurance (Germany), tax-funded care allowances (Austria) and tax-funded in-kind services (Sweden and Norway). Although there are challenges to be overcome to boost participation in private long-term care insurance markets, these are now growing in France and the United States.

Notes

1. These projections, based on data from 18 OECD countries, assume current age-related cost patterns hold over time and that spending is unaffected by other factors.

2. Changes in social arrangements have resulted in more frail and elderly people living alone or only with an elderly spouse. Changes in the size and employment status of the working age population appear to have reduced the potential for family care of frail older people. An increasingly better-informed and better-educated population expects to receive basic social protection against catastrophic costs of intensive care needs as well as a broader range of services of better quality.

3. The boundary between health care and long-term care is difficult to draw and is drawn differently across countries. Hence, it is difficult to disentangle the two in expenditure data.

4. To offset the incentive under open-ended fee-for-service reimbursement for individual physicians to increase volume, some countries have experimented with regulated fee schedules where physicians are reimbursed on the basis of points per service and the value of a point is determined according to the volume of services delivered by physicians during the reference period to keep total expenditures within a global budget.

5. In Eastern Europe, prices and wages in the health sector remain low and under-the-table gratuity payments to providers are common.

6. Over the past three decades, there has been a general convergence across the OECD in the share of spending represented by the public sector, in that it tended to decline in many countries with the highest share of spending (e.g. Czech Republic, Norway, United Kingdom) and increase in countries with the lowest share (e.g. Greece, Turkey, United States) (OECD, 2003c).

7. For a review of the evidence, see Docteur and Oxley (2003).

8. This is an unweighted average for the 23 OECD countries for which data or estimates are available (see Table 2.1). The average excludes Belgium, Greece, Poland, Portugal, Sweden, Turkey, and the United Kingdom. If the United States, in which private health insurance constitutes 35% of health spending, is excluded, the average drops to 5.9%.

9. Between 1990 and 2000, private health insurance financing grew as a share of total health expenditure in certain OECD countries (e.g. Canada, Germany and New Zealand). In other countries, however, the importance of private health insurance in funding total and private health expenditures has decreased (e.g. Austria, Ireland and Australia).

10. The Netherlands plans to move to a system of mandatory private health insurance for the entire population with public guarantees to offset possible negative effects. These include an obligation for insurers to accept all applicants; a prohibition on differentiating premiums according to age or health status; a governmentally defined basic insurance package; income-related tax refunds to increase equity of financing; and redistribution of premiums according to the level of risk borne by each insurer.

11. Under Medicare+ Choice, beneficiaries of the public Medicare programme can enrol in a managed-care plan or other privately administered health insurance plan. These plans are paid a set fee per beneficiary per month. Because financing is predominantly public, the model cannot be termed private health insurance according to the definition used by the OECD.

12. Health represents the largest share of GDP in the United States, Switzerland and Germany, and these countries are also among the top five countries in terms of per-capita spending levels (OECD, 2003d).

13. In the United States, administrative costs account for 31% of spending on health care, as compared to 16.7% in Canada (Woolhandler *et al.*, 2003). Overhead costs for US health insurance companies were 11.7% of health care spending, compared with 1.3% in Canada's public-contract system and 3.6% in the US Medicare programme.

14. Public integrated models spend little on transaction costs and may well have overhead costs below those in Canada (Himmelstein and Woolhandler, 1986).

15. The limited available evidence is reviewed in OECD (2004c).

16. For instance, as discussed earlier, systems with multiple payers may require additional resources to cover administrative costs, as compared with single-payer systems.

ISBN 92-64-01555-8
Towards High-Performing Health Systems
© OECD 2004

Chapter 5

Increasing value for money
in health systems:
the quest for efficiency

Over the long term, improvements in efficiency may be the only way – certainly the most appealing way – of reconciling rising demands for health care with public financing constraints. A primary current focus of OECD countries, therefore, is on achieving greater value for money from their health-care systems. Cross-country data suggest that there are inefficiencies in health systems that provide scope for improvements in the cost-effectiveness of health-care delivery and increased productivity. In addition, the economics of the health sector, typically characterised by market failures and heavy public intervention, suggest a high risk of excess or misallocated spending that results in waste. Many of the initiatives recently undertaken as part of efforts to improve health or the quality of health care may prove to be cost-effective ones over the longer term or even in the short run. In addition, a number of other approaches geared at reducing waste (administrative or other) or improving productivity are also possible.

Evidence of inefficiency in health systems

The significant differences seen across countries in the capacity of health systems, the resources expended, the volumes and types of services furnished and the health outcomes attained, suggests that there is variation across systems in efficiency. Various characteristics and complexities of health systems that cause them to function in ways not likely to lead to optimal outcomes suggest that the scope for efficiency improvements may be quite significant. Among the most important such characteristics are information asymmetries, uncertainty as to needs and appropriateness in health care, and poorly aligned economic incentives.

For example, many studies have documented widespread variation in the use of technologies and treatments both across and within OECD countries. This variation, which may be due to different economic incentives, technology adoption or diffusion policies, or other factors, suggests that there is also variation in the cost-effectiveness of use. An illustration of the differences in the use made of particular treatments can be seen in the great discrepancy between the incidence of heart disease, as measured through cause-of-death data, and rates in use of surgical interventions (Figures 5.1 and 5.2). Cross-country research has found that the relationship between heart disease incidence and use of revascularisation procedures is a weak one (Moïse, 2003).

Such variation probably indicates under-performance of some health-care systems. Health systems in some countries may be missing chances to provide treatments that would benefit patients. Others could be using more treatments than are optimal, if some of the treatments performed are not clinically indicated. Higher than optimal treatment rates may also occur, even if all of the treatments provide some clinical benefit, if countries are investing at points beyond which they attain diminishing marginal returns to investment. Ensuring that systems deliver evidence-based medicine will, therefore, not only result in better care, but it may very well result in less costly care.

Further study is required to better understand the implications of various levels of resource use and treatment rates on health outcomes. Nevertheless, evidence from an international study of heart-attack care suggests that differences across countries in rate

Figure 5.1. **Ischaemic heart disease, total population, age standardised mortality rate, 2000**

Figure 5.2. **Coronary re-vascularisation procedures[1] per 100 000 population, 2000**

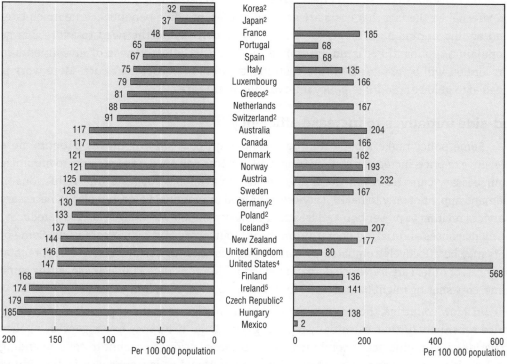

1. Coronary artery bypass grafts (CABG) and percutaneous coronary interventions conducted on an inpatient basis.
2. Procedure data not available.
3. Data are from 1999.
4. CABG data from 1999.
5. CABG data from 2001.

Source: OECD Health Data 2003.

of outcome improvements are much more modest than the differences in treatment trends, suggesting scope for improving cost-effectiveness of care (McClellan and Kessler, 2003). Evidence from that study suggested declining marginal benefit from intensive use of technology for heart-attack care. While the question of whether additional investment that results in marginal improvement is "worth the cost" is a matter of judgement, such cross-country studies can be useful in shedding light on the implications of various choices.

Cost-effectiveness of investment in disease prevention and health promotion

Governments looking for ways to increase the value for money from expenditure on health may review the overall balance between public spending on health promotion (or disease prevention) and spending on health care. In most OECD countries, spending on health care accounts for more than 90% of total health spending, while spending on health promotion activities represents less than 5% of the total (OECD, 2003d). Therefore, a superficially persuasive idea is that governments are spending too much on curative medicine and could greatly enhance the efficiency of their health systems and save public resources if they put more emphasis on prevention and early detection.

There is strong evidence as to the cost-effectiveness of interventions to tackle communicable diseases, such as vaccination and immunisation and, by-and-large, this evidence is acted upon in OECD countries. However, there is often a lack of evidence on the cost-effectiveness of measures to prevent non-communicable diseases, partly because the time lags between interventions and results can be very protracted, which makes it difficult to establish cause and effect. Where there is cost-effectiveness evidence, this will be affected by the fact that costs are accrued at present while benefits accrue much later and are discounted accordingly. Given the lags involved and the need to address large population groups, there is no assurance that the cost-effectiveness of investments in prevention will be greater than the cost-effectiveness of subsequent cure. More work is needed to guide appropriate policy intervention in this area.

Demand-side initiatives to increase efficiency

Some policy makers hope that because patient cost-sharing makes patients more sensitive to price, increasing cost-sharing requirements will encourage patients to minimize unnecessary care. However, the limited evidence available suggests that reductions in demand apply not only to health services of limited or marginal value, but also to necessary services relating to prevention and treatment (Siu *et al.*, 1986; Manning *et al.*, 1987), reducing early diagnoses and risking poorer future health outcomes and higher care costs. Some of this may be effectively combated by eliminating cost sharing for preventive care, prenatal services, or other care for which demand reductions are considered undesirable. At the same time, cost-sharing might be increased for services considered of limited value.

In a few countries, there is interest in the potential to take the approach of increasing price-sensitivity further, essentially replacing first-dollar insurance coverage with a policy covering catastrophic needs combined with a personal savings account to cover spending on health services. Experimentation with such approaches is under way in the United States. The approach faces an array of challenges, ranging from the potential risk-segmentation problem (which undermines the pooling effect of insurance) inherent in a choice-based system to limited consumer demand due to risk aversion.

However, it also appears there is scope for better communication of evidence on best practices to patients, taking advantage of trends toward more active consumerism in health care. Some initiatives in this direction are evident. For example, in the United States, interactive computer software has been developed that allows patients to better understand optional treatments for conditions such as benign prostatic hyperplasia and breast cancer, and to furnish customized information on the likelihood of various outcomes. Patients, as compared with their physicians, may be more inclined to choose less invasive and intensive forms of treatment when fully informed as to risks and likely outcomes.

Some health systems employ mechanisms geared towards steering or influencing patient demand for health services. For example, several countries make use of so-called gatekeeper physicians, general practitioners who regulate access to specialist care, who may also face financial incentives to influence how care is directed. Also used are requirements to obtain second opinions or pre-authorisation before using certain services (surgery, specialist care, emergency-room care), or even counselling services, such as nurse practitioners who staff telephone inquiry lines. All of these approaches offer potential to improve the cost-effectiveness of care, although depending on how they are employed, they may conflict with responsiveness goals and may add to administrative cost.

Supply-side initiatives to increase efficiency

Given the extent to which health-care purchasers and suppliers act as decision-making agents for individual consumers and patients, supply-side initiatives probably hold the greatest promise for efficiency improvements. A wide range of changes have been made to the way in which health services are organised, financed, and delivered with the aim of making systems more efficient.[1] Notably, in many OECD countries in which both financing and delivery of health care are a public responsibility, there has been effort to create more distinction between the purchasing and providing functions, so as to better replicate the conditions under which normal economic transactions occur. Such changes, where they have been made, have generally, though not always, been viewed as successful. Less clear is the experience with decentralisation of public health-care decision-making and administration. Here, many countries (e.g. Spain) have taken steps towards decentralisation. Some have been viewed as successful, but not all have retained these changes. Finding the right balance in terms of central and decentralised decision-making has proved challenging and what is appropriate is likely to vary across countries. Among other important reforms are efforts to uncover fraud and abuse in health systems and efforts to integrate health-care delivery on a horizontal or vertical basis so as to benefit from economies of scale or opportunities for reducing redundancy and waste. Of particular promise are efforts to integrate health and long-term care services, and efforts to improve continuity of care across the full episode of treatment, which may involve multiple service providers. Because such reforms tend to be context-specific, it is difficult to generalise about their effects, but it is clear that there are good success stories worthy of study (see Box 5.1).

Efficient deployment of human resources for health care

To deploy the health workforce efficiently, policy makers must take into account critical factors influencing efficiency, including the implications of various methods of payment and mixes of skill levels. Whether efficiency has improved in the ambulatory care sector over

---

Box 5.1. **Recent efficiency improvements by the US Veterans Health Administration**

The reform of the US Veterans Health Administration (VHA) serves as an example of a successful re-engineering of a government-owned and operated health-care system (Kizer, 2000). The VHA, created to finance and provide medical and rehabilitation care to disabled and indigent military veterans, saw itself confronted with numerous reports on operational and managerial failures and deteriorating public image in the early 1990s and competition from the private sector. This crisis lead to a major restructuring effort with the implementation of universal primary care and the creation of integrated service networks, which aggregated all VHA providers in a given area into one unit, starting in the mid-1990s. Combined with a measurement-based performance management program, investment in information technology and use of clinical guidelines, those innovations led to substantial improvements in quality of care. Within four years, surgical mortality fell by 9% and compliance with accepted preventive care standards rose from 34% to 81% (Khuri et al., 1998; Kizer, 2000).[1] At the same time, estimated per patient costs fell by 25% in a five-year period, showing that cost reduction and quality improvement can occur together (Kizer, 2000).

1. One hospital in the Department of Veterans Affairs uses hand-held, wireless computer technology and bar-coding, which has cut overall hospital medication error rates by 70% (Agency for Healthcare Research and Quality, 2000).

Figure 5.3. **Doctor consultations per capita, 2000**

Figure 5.4. **Change in number of doctor consultations per capita, 1990 to 2000**

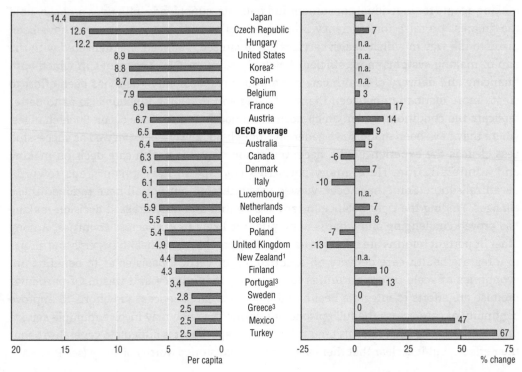

Note: The OECD average change excludes Germany, Hungary, Ireland, Korea, Luxembourg, New Zealand, Norway, the Slovak Republic, Spain, Switzerland and the United States. Data for Denmark include consultations by telephone, but exclude consultations with specialists. The Netherlands do not include contacts for maternal and childcare, nor discharge planning visits in hospitals and nursing homes. Portugal and Turkey exclude visits to private practitioners. The UK does not include consultations with specialists in the independent sector or consultations with specialists outside hospital outpatient departments. The US estimates include all telephone calls for medical advice, prescriptions and test results; they are therefore not limited to physician visits.
1. 2001.
2. 1999.
3. 1998.
Source: OECD Health Data 2003.

time is not clear, although there are very large differences across countries in structure and performance of the health-care workforces. For example, in 2000, there were very large differences across countries in the number of consultations with doctors per capita (Figure 5.3). The average across OECD countries was 6.5 visits per person per year (OECD, 2003c). It ranged from a low of less than three visits per person per year in Turkey, Mexico, Greece and Sweden, to over ten visits per year in Japan, the Czech Republic and Hungary. Over the past decade, the rate of consultations has increased slightly in most OECD countries for which data are available, with notable exceptions, such as the United Kingdom, where doctor consultations dropped by 13% during that period (Figure 5.4).

Payment methods can influence productivity in ambulatory care

There is considerable variation within and across OECD countries in physician payment methods. Some systems that fund health care through taxation employ general practitioners directly and pay them a salary (*e.g.* Greece, Portugal, Spain and Sweden), whereas in Australia, Denmark, New Zealand, Norway and the United Kingdom, general practitioners are self-employed and are paid by a mix of capitation, salary and fee-for-service. General practitioners in insurance-based health-care systems such as Austria, Belgium, France, Germany, Japan, Korea and Switzerland tend to be independent contractors who are mainly paid on a fee-for-service basis. Ambulatory-care specialists are generally paid either by salary or fee-for-service, with salary payment being more common in the public sector.

The available evidence provides only limited information on the impact of payment method on physician activity levels. Fee-for-service payments to physicians seem to increase the quantity of medical services, but reduce rates of referral and the volume of prescriptions as compared to payment by capitation or salary (Gosden *et al.*, 1999 and 2001). However, the Norwegian experience of operating two remuneration systems side-by-side for a period of time demonstrates that physician practice patterns are influenced not only by payment methods, but also by clinical factors and influence by peers.

Countries' experiences have revealed the adverse incentives of simple payment methods. It has been argued that fee-for-service payments to providers, combined with no controls on the services actually delivered, might lead to high prices, high rates of unnecessary service utilisation and rising expenditures. Under a capitated or salaried system, concerns have been raised that physicians may find it financially rewarding to furnish fewer services or select people with fewer health needs or actively discourage high-risk people ("cream-skimming").

To counteract the adverse incentives of individual payment methods, some public and private payers have moved from paying physicians by a simple method towards more sophisticated payment systems that integrate caps on expenditure, control of fee levels, and health-care utilisation reviews in addition to a combination of payment by capitation or salary and payment by fee-for-service. Blended-payment methods that combine a fixed component through either capitation or salary and a variable component through fee-for-service for specific cost-effective interventions, such as those used for general practitioners in the United Kingdom, may produce a desirable mix of incentives. However, in practice they also pose challenges. For example, Germany is one of several countries in which regulated fees are combined with limits on the total value of payments. Because such approaches encourage individual physicians to increase service volume in order to maintain income levels, regional physician associations in Germany monitor service volume and penalize physicians whose high service volumes cannot be attributed to case mix.

The appropriate skill mix

The ratio of physicians to nurses varies greatly across OECD member countries, raising questions as to whether countries are adopting an appropriate skill mix between physicians and nurses in the delivery of health care. Countries' skill-mix arrangements likely depend on productivity considerations, health worker and patient preferences, and contextual, economic and social factors. There is some evidence suggesting that certain tasks traditionally performed by physicians could be transferred to highly qualified nurses, such as nurse practitioners, without significant changes in the quality of care provided. In fact, such changes are being made in some countries. For example, in the United States, nurse practitioners in some states increasingly provide services that are also provided by primary care physicians (such as check-ups and gynaecological examinations), in some cases acting as extenders of a physician-based practice. Appropriate changes in the skill mix of health professionals have the potential to reduce personnel costs, improve labour productivity and lessen the constraints that result from shortages in specific types of staff.

Improving efficiency in the hospital sector

The hospital sector is one in which significant efficiency improvements have been made in many OECD countries. Between 1985 and 2000, for instance, the average length of an acute-care hospital stay declined from 9.6 to 6.5 days. Of course, shorter stays are not necessarily more cost-effective, particularly if short stays are more service-intensive and equally costly, or if health outcomes suffer. But member countries have not documented problems with respect to the latter concern.[2] Other evidence of improved efficiency includes the general long-term trend towards decline in capacity, as measured by number of beds, even as the number of hospital admissions has increased in several countries (OECD, 2003c). And there has been a shift across countries to the use of day surgery, made technically feasible by medical innovations such as laparoscopy, which permits less invasive procedures.

Waiting times for elective surgery may, in some respects, be considered an efficiency indicator, although it may be interpreted in different ways. For any given elective surgery rate there may well be optimum waiting times that are above zero. Although patients, who may be disabled or in pain from their conditions, will generally prefer earlier treatment, and there are likely to be other social costs incurred by excessive waiting, there can also be considerable savings in reduced surgical capacity, and hence lower unit costs, from forming queues. That arises from the stochastic nature of the demand for emergency surgical and medical care. Assuming a system is operating at a high level of productivity, a queue of elective patients helps to ensure that hospital capacity can be kept occupied when the rate of emergency admissions (which must be given priority) fluctuates.

Two policy questions drive today's continuing efforts to improve efficiency in the hospital sector. First, what sorts of changes can be undertaken to reduce waste, improve cost-efficiency, or increase productivity in hospital care? Countries investigating possibilities for efficiency improvements have diverse outstanding concerns relating to appropriateness of surgical procedures, fraud and abuse, and administration and management decision-making. Second, what sorts of economic and administrative incentives are effective in motivating efficiency improvements? With respect to both questions, there is much to learn from recent experience, as well as much room for further experimentation and study.

Enhancing managerial capacity and independence and cost accountability of hospitals

Many hospital systems, particularly those run by a national health system, have faced tight budget limits with little management freedom. A number of management- and budget-related reforms have aimed at improving the incentives for efficiency within individual hospitals. For example, budget periods have been lengthened beyond one year to discourage providers from spending up to the budget ceiling at the end of each budget year, while hospitals have been allowed to keep any budget savings. In many countries, capital is allocated independently from current budgets and the cost of capital is not integrated into the budget process. In contrast, the United Kingdom and New Zealand introduced arrangements under which hospitals are charged a rate of return on capital invested in order to encourage a more parsimonious use of capital. Countries that have embarked on purchaser-provider separation have usually granted more autonomy to public hospital managers. In some cases, the granting of autonomy has been linked to performance i.e. "earned autonomy" – giving hospitals more managerial independence, and allowing greater flexibility and experimentation in resource allocation within each hospital. The public-sector nature of the labour force has often placed limits on the extent of managerial flexibility. Competitive tendering has been introduced for support services in public hospitals (and many other public services) in some countries, with evidence of cost savings for a given level of quality (Domberger and Jensen, 1997).

Evolution of payment methods to reward productivity

The arrangements formerly used to pay hospitals in many OECD countries have not encouraged efficiency and sometimes had the opposite effect – for example, where costs were fully reimbursed *ex post*. Many fee-for-service price schedules poorly reflect underlying costs, often because they have not appropriately allowed for technological change and falling prices of equipment. Prospective, case-related payment systems, such as those employing diagnosis related groups (DRGs) to set, in advance of service provision, payments based on the estimated cost of hospital care for a particular episode, appear to provide a more effective framework for administered pricing. These have the additional advantage of inducing hospitals to reduce the costs per care episode.

Activity-based systems require careful judgements about the relative costs of treating different conditions and the payments need to be set at levels that just cover the average cost of supply by an efficient provider, something that is extremely difficult to achieve in practice.[3] Furthermore, for access or quality reasons, policy makers may wish to subsidise providers whose services are higher cost, as with rural hospitals that may have relatively low service volumes and hospitals that provide specialised care for very high-risk patients. Like any price schedule, prospective payment amounts also need to be adjusted regularly to take into account the impact of changing technology and other factors on relative costs and prices.

Activity-based payment systems can induce increased supply, a positive outcome where there are waiting lists and unused productivity reserves that can be drawn upon. However, payers need to be vigilant about adverse incentive effects. With a fixed payment per hospital episode, hospitals have an incentive to discharge patients as early as possible, to upgrade patients into more costly diagnostic groups and to "cream-skim" to avoid costly patients. These problems may require some re-balancing of the risks of significantly higher costs for individual patients between the purchaser and the provider, and a variety of mixed systems have been proposed to achieve this[4] (van Barneveld *et al.*, 2001).

Prospective payments systems can lead to budget over-runs as a result of the increased supply of services. The move to a DRG-type system within the context of competing hospital units in the Stockholm area of Sweden in the early 1990s was aborted: even though there were important increases in output and reductions in waiting times, budget overruns were large enough to require corrective action (Forsberg *et al.*, 2001). Austria and some other countries have attempted to resolve this dilemma by imposing an overall budget, with the budget envelope allocated to individual hospitals based on their activity levels over the budgetary period. Incentives to increase output may be blunted if providers foresee that the fruits of their increased efforts are likely to be clawed back through lower payments per unit, especially if values fall below variable cost. However, in cases of existing excess supply of health-care services and no waiting lists, such arrangements can encourage supply-driven demand.[5]

Role of price competition in driving efficiency improvements in the hospital sector

Widespread competition in the supply of health care already exists in a number of areas; for example, in primary care, where doctors compete for clients and where there is widespread consumer choice. Competition also exists in the hospital sector in many countries where individuals can choose their hospital, although they may be in no position to "shop around" when they require emergency care. However, competition in terms of price is limited and, with the exception of the private insurance sector in the United States, prices are generally set through negotiations of a bilateral monopoly nature between the payers and providers, grouped together.

A limited number of countries have experimented with price competition – as opposed to imposing uniform price schedules – between providers as a means of inducing efficiency improvements. Competition in markets for private health-care services – driven by competition among insurers in the United States – appears to have contributed to slower growth, temporarily, in health-care costs. Elsewhere, experiments to create health-care markets for clinical services in public systems have run into a range of problems – whether related more to the market structure of the health-care system or more to opposition on the part of the professional monopolies is unclear – and have sometimes been abandoned. Selected problems are: lack of excess capacity, together with waiting lists for elective care (such that hospitals are not able to bid for extra work); lack of management skills for operating in competitive markets; absence of skilled third-party payers or purchasers combined with continued central control over purchasing decisions; high transaction costs (difficult to justify to a sceptical public); concerns about local access to care (governments cannot allow hospitals to close suddenly, especially where they are the only local supplier); difficulty in setting prices that appropriately reflect resource costs where competition is weak; and resistance from the professional health-care workers (especially doctors and nurses) with monopoly power who have "captured" some aspects of the supply of publicly owned health care.

Improving efficiency in delivery of long-term care

A number of measures have been adopted as part of efforts to increase efficiency in long-term care delivery. Among the most commonly used approaches are:

- Pre-admission screening to nursing homes wherever possible, to ensure that only those for whom this is the only practicable alternative enter an expensive care institution.

- Greater definition in setting public subsidies for long-term care, to enable packages of care in and out of institutions to be more finely graduated to the patient's needs.

- Allowing payment for home care services as an alternative to institutionalisation, with a focus on intensive packages that represent a real alternative to a nursing home.

- Greater care management, in which the patient's case is kept under review and changes in care services recommended when their circumstances change.

- Earlier intervention to support family care-givers, *e.g.* with counselling, respite care, and help with heavy duty tasks, rather than waiting until the care-giver cannot continue and a nursing home may be the only prospect.

All of these measures feature to some degree in the system of long-term care insurance introduced in Japan in 2000, and some have also been implemented in countries such as Australia, Canada, the Netherlands, the United Kingdom and the United States. However, there is considerable scope for such measures to be introduced more widely in these and other countries. It remains a too-common experience for patients and their families that the delivery of care remains uncoordinated, with insufficient collaboration between care professionals in different sectors.

Steps have been taken in a number of countries to improve the interaction between the acute and long-term care health sectors, for example, through introducing multi-disciplinary assessment teams, and by aligning the financial signals to ensure that patients who now need long-term care do not remain in hospital. It is important to ensure that such efforts result in delivery of more appropriate care in a more appropriate setting; otherwise, apparent gains in the hospital sector may result in a less efficient system overall.

Promoting efficient use of health technology

Technological advances can increase efficiency in health care. Using US data, Cutler and McClellan (2001) concluded that the total benefits of changes in technology exceeded the corresponding costs for at least four of the conditions over the period studied (findings for breast cancer were equivocal). Although the study did not address whether similar benefits could have accrued from less costly investments, it found a clear and consistent association between more intensive treatment and better outcomes. Other work suggests that cross-country differences in outcomes, at least for heart attack care, are much more modest than differences in treatment trends (McClellan and Kessler, 2003).

Given the role of health-related technology as the primary factor contributing to health cost growth, better management of technology has been recognized by policy makers as an important frontier for efficiency improvements. Nevertheless, given the role of technology in contributing to improvements in health outcomes, it is important that management efforts proceed carefully.

Prospects for increasing efficiency in the pharmaceutical sector

The pharmaceutical sector now accounts for an average of over 16% of total health expenditure in OECD countries, a share that has grown by 1.6 percentage points over the past decade. The number of new drugs increased considerably in recent years, and the movement towards new, more expensive products has been one of the main driving forces in increasing pharmaceutical expenditure. This growth has thus contributed to the increase in overall health spending although, to some extent, medicines may be substituting for surgical or other treatments, resulting in more growth in this sector relative to others.

Administered payment systems, which are common features of health systems in OECD countries, have special challenges when it comes to pharmaceuticals. Socially optimally prices need to take into account not only the value of the specific medicine, but also the costs of research and development, if future innovation is to be sustained. The basic science supporting pharmaceuticals and other health-related technologies is frequently carried out in publicly funded institutions such as the National Institutes for Health in the United States and the CNRS in France. However, the cost of converting a scientific understanding to a new remedy, and increasingly the cost of the underlying scientific research, is borne by the private sector.[6] This work is largely financed through the rents to successful innovations conferred through patent protection.

Innovative pharmaceutical products are frequently subject to patent protection, whose purpose is to confer temporary monopoly rights to reward innovation. However, the rewards to patent holders are limited by the price purchasers are willing to pay. National insurance authorities often limit the price at which they will reimburse patented products, and in some countries there are direct controls on the prices at which patented products can be marketed. In aggregate, these cost-control measures reduce the global revenues of producers, and result in significant disparities between the prices received between one country and another. Such practices can discourage innovation by reducing the returns to investment in drugs.

For products no longer under patent protection, lowering costs through market competition is increasingly encouraged. Laws have been passed to allow the substitution of generic equivalents for prescriptions which nominate brand-name products. To give consumers an incentive to demand such substitution, insurance reimbursements are often limited to the lowest "reference price" in a pharmaceutical class. Such approaches offer genuine prospects for increasing efficiency in the use of prescription drugs. However, manufacturers, therapists and patients often protest that such policies are unfair because the "reference product" may not be appropriate for all patients. It can also inhibit the diffusion of new treatments by making them unaffordable to those reliant on social insurance to finance their treatment. Facilitating availability and use of generic alternatives can avert these negative effects by fostering price competition at the level of the molecule, rather than the therapeutic class.

To the extent that such pricing systems result in lower returns on investment in research and development in the pharmaceutical industry, such systems may reduce incentives for innovation. On the other hand, if employed appropriately, reference pricing may instead direct incentives for innovation to development of drugs that are notable break-throughs, rather than modest modifications of existing formulas (Pammoli and Riccaboni, 2004).[7] This may in turn contribute to a net welfare gain. In addition, all stakeholders are likely to agree that, if policy makers deem public cost-containment to be necessary in the pharmaceutical sector, reference-pricing schemes are preferable to approaches that would make across-the-board cuts in public financing without taking into account alternative treatments.

Health technology assessment as a tool to increase efficiency in health-care delivery

Health technology assessment (HTA) and pharmaco-economic assessment are playing an increasing role in many OECD countries. Such assessments are a form of evaluation in which information on a technology (or an application) and its impacts is produced, synthesised and appraised in a process designed to facilitate evidence-based decision making. Effectiveness is taken into account, as may be cost-effectiveness, effectiveness relative to existing technology, and relevant legal, social, or ethical issues.

Assessments are used in some countries to help decision makers in pricing and reimbursement decisions under public programmes. Governments are increasingly requiring pharmaco-economic assessments of the costs and benefits of new drugs, in addition to evidence on their safety, before they can be sold or listed as reimbursable by public insurers (Dickson *et al.*, 2003). Assessments are also used in the development of evidence-based clinical practice guidelines and performance standards, both of which can be used to increase efficiency in health-care delivery. Health technology assessment can be used to support decision making at the micro (clinical), meso (hospital or health authority) and macro (government, insurance) levels.

The role of HTA is highly valued by decision makers and this only likely to increase. HTA is valuable because many widely used and funded technologies are of uncertain effect in terms of improving patient health (Fuchs, 1987; Maynard *et al.*, 2000).[8] Furthermore, the rapid pace of innovation and publication of new studies result in decision makers having difficulties in keeping up with the large volume of evidence on the impact of technologies.[9] Finally, many OECD health systems have diffused decision-making process closer to the patient and as a result there will be more decision-makers requiring access to high-quality evidence.

There has been little systematic evidence on the impact HTA has had on decision making, health system functioning or on health outcomes.[10] However, a number of initiatives could result in greater impact, including broadening the focus of assessment, assess older as well as new technologies, make better use of information and communication technologies, take steps to increase the reliability of results and to enhance trust in them; increase targeted dissemination activities; and improve methodologies to take into account patient values (OECD, 2004d).

Further, there is a need to improve the interaction between producers and users of HTA. For example, early dialogue between the users and producers would facilitate collection of relevant and timely evidence that takes into account the specific characteristics of the technology and the particular questions that are relevant to the decision maker (OECD, 2004d). There is also a need to ensure that the production of HTA information is attuned to the particular institutional features of the health system, and in particular to the decision-making bodies within those systems. Box 5.2 provides an overview of how HTA and the decision-making processes have been adapted to the needs and institutional characteristics of three OECD health systems.

It is increasingly recognised that access to high quality evidence is a necessary, but not a sufficient, condition to manage the uptake and use of health technologies effectively. The decision-making process itself is an important part of successfully using evidence and implementing recommendations. For example, decisions made in a transparent manner, based on evidence and incorporates an appeals mechanism are far more likely to have wider stakeholder support (OECD, 2004d).

It is also important recognise that HTA can inform decision making but it is not a substitute for it. Values, culture, ethics, psychology and politics will, and should, complicate the equation. The optimal integration of scientific evidence with transparent processes in which evidence can be interpreted is a complex issue. The National Institute of Clinical Excellence in the UK is a recognised leader in the field and its methodologies for appraising evidence have set international benchmarks (Hill *et al.* 2003).

Since the introduction of HTA in the seventies, significant advances have been made in the production and use of evidence in decision-making. Many challenges remain, including those that future technologies may also pose to decision makers and assessors. Over the next 20 years, genetic engineering, tissue engineering, and other areas of biotechnology will take health beyond the traditional treatment concepts of palliation, cure and prevention and toward a new concept of enhancement, one of improving human performance. Prospects include enhancements to memory, cognitive processing, and physical capacity. Such new technologies may have the ability to reduce personal side-effects, but will at the same time have important economic and bioethical consequences (Moldrup *et al.*, 2003).

Policy tools to manage the diffusion of new health-related technology

OECD countries have used a variety of approaches to manage the diffusion of health-related technologies, including regulatory controls, positive and negative lists and prospective payment mechanisms. However, in many instances these tools can be blunt and have unintended consequences. In recent years, many countries have employed policy tools that aim to take value into account in managing health-related technology. The following set of policy tools, while not exhaustive, provides some useful examples of innovative mechanisms intended to foster optimal integration of new health technologies into health-care delivery.

Box 5.2. **Use of health technology assessment in decision-making in three OECD health systems**

Access to high-quality and trusted evidence that is relevant to the decision maker's needs is essential if health technology assessment (HTA) is to play a role in decision making. At the same time, decision-making processes themselves need to facilitate the use of evidence and HTA. The following three examples show how HTA is being facilitated and used in three health systems, with varying institutional responsibilities for decision making.

Australia

In Australia, health technology assessment (HTA) has had its greatest impact on two federal health services financing programmes: the Medicare Benefits Scheme (MBS) and the Pharmaceutical Benefits Scheme (PBS). Both of these programmes require i) mandatory economic evaluation of potential new benefits, ii) appraisal of evidence by the relevant advisory committees, and iii) decisions made by the minister based on the committees' recommendations. The production and use of HTA have developed over time to meet the needs of the two programmes, and have resulted in the development of influential guidelines on economic evaluations and in highly focused and relevant HTA activities. However, HTA has been more limited in terms of its influence on clinical practice.

While HTA processes are generally accepted and supported by stakeholders in Australia, the outcomes of decisions influenced by HTA can be controversial with industry and medical professional bodies. A review of 355 PBS applications shows that the Pharmaceutical Benefits Advisory Committee rejected 25% of initial applications.

Canada

In Canada, HTA activities have devolved along provincial lines and coordinated through the Canadian Coordinating Office of HTA (CCOHTA). In a devolved health care system, one of the major challenges in Canada has been to improve the use of HTA in decision-making. In response to this challenge, the Ontario Health Technology Advisory Committee was established to bring together senior hospital decision makers and clinical experts to identify new and emerging technologies and set priorities for assessment. The committee promotes the use of HTA in decision making by bridging the worlds of evidence and decision-making. Under this model, early assessments or evaluations of technology are based on the characteristics of the technology, the evidence available, and the needs of decision makers. For example, when possible, the Ministry aims to complete a HTA within a 12-week period. The Ontario model is a systematic bottom-up method of incorporating evidence into decision making. Whilst the programme has only recently been implemented, it will be important to evaluate its impact on decision-making and use of HTA evidence in the future.

Mexico

Mexico has a complex health care system, with multiple levels of public and private decision making. Whilst it has the capacity to conduct HTA, its main challenge is to create coordinating mechanisms between institutions to facilitate HTA use in decision making.

To promote HTA use in decision making, the Mexican Ministry of Health recently established institutional support for HTA through the Center for Technological Excellence to develop national policies for HTA. Meanwhile, the Mexican Institute of Social Security-IMSS (the main public body responsible for providing health care delivery to almost 50 million Mexicans) is responsible for conducting HTA and for creating mechanisms to facilitate the use of HTA in decision making. At the policy level, it develops policies that incorporate those new medical technologies that optimise service capacity. At the health-care facility level, it develops information systems and management tools. At the clinical level, it develops clinical guidelines.

The initiative has had an impact on decision making. For example, it has facilitated efficient resource allocation decisions of new technologies and radio surgery services, based on information supplied by a registry of the functional status of medical equipment.

Source: Duran and Coburn (2003).

Cost, volume, and value agreements

Cost, volume and value agreements are commonly used to shift and control costs. Under Australia's fee-for-service Medicare programme, for example, price-volume agreements have been implemented for pathology, diagnostic imaging, and anaesthetics. In effect, the government and professional groups agree that expenditure will be limited to a certain amount over a period of three to five years. If utilisation exceeds expectations, prices go down. When new technologies are funded, allowed expenditures are increased; however, the cap is re-fixed at that point. This provides certainty as to outlays, despite the formally uncapped nature of the financing arrangements.

Some such agreements aim to take into account the value of technology, but this is an imprecise art. In the United Kingdom, for example, an agreement between government, industry, providers and other stakeholders was reached on the purchase and provision of Beta Interferon in the treatment of multiple sclerosis. Under this scheme, if an agreed level of effectiveness was not achieved, the government and manufacturer would renegotiate the price of the drug (UK Department of Health, 2002). Such mechanisms can increase cost-effectiveness and promote access to new technology while information is gathered, and encourage the manufacturer to promote appropriate prescribing.

Payment mechanisms

Payment mechanisms can act as powerful incentives to deliver technologies in line with perceived health needs and evidence. For example, the so-called Immunise Australia Plan, launched in 1997, included a range of financial incentives to general practitioners as well as payments to parents that helped attain significant rises in immunisation rates. Some US policy makers hoped that the combination of economic incentives and management tools available to managed-care plans in the United States would result in more cost-effective use of health technology, but evidence as to whether that occurred is mixed.[11]

Planning agreements

Planning agreements between various stakeholders, including national and provincial governments, can be used to set diffusion guidelines. Such agreements enable the central agency, for example, to set key objectives and help diffuse technologies in line with these objectives. In Austria, national and regional decision makers have agreed to a plan to expand diffusion of PET (positron emission tomography) machines beyond the current level over a set period of time. The plan takes into account level of clinical need, population distribution and geographic equity of access.

Implementation programmes

Implementation programmes appear effective in appropriately diffusing technologies where there are wider service implications, as examples from the Netherlands and Norway demonstrate. In the Netherlands, following six regional pilot tests of stroke services, the government commenced a national stroke-service implementation programme. A working group developed service guidelines as well as a comprehensive strategy for their implementation in 23 regions. Implementation is in progress, with early signs of success. The Norwegian National Centre for Telemedicine is a resource centre that gathers, produces and provides information about telemedicine. It supplies research, development and advisory services to assist the Norwegian Health Service in implementing telemedicine services. It has an active research programme that pilots and evaluates new projects before diffusion. It also examines future technologies, applications, and service models that may bear on future health service delivery.

Co-operation amongst service providers

Enhancing co-operation amongst providers and health-care organisations may reduce pressures to minimise prices that could otherwise be generated through competition; however, it appears to be associated with lower rates of capital-intensive acquisitions (Pritchard, 2002). Co-operation also appears to be major success factor in multidisciplinary service provision. Examples of such services include hospital-in-the-home programmes and stroke services. These types of services require seamless service provision from a wide array of providers found in the ambulatory, acute and community sectors. Co-operation amongst these providers has been found to be vital to the success of such programmes.

The role of private health insurance in efficiency improvements

A significant part of the appeal of private health insurance is its potential to improve the efficiency of health-care delivery. Its ability to meet that potential is believed to depend largely on the ability to attain a marketplace in which value-based competition occurs. However, experience to date shows not only that there are serious challenges to be overcome in achieving competition on such grounds, but furthermore it is not entirely clear that competition amongst insurers is either necessary or sufficient to drive efficiency improvements.

Efforts by private health insurers to increase cost-effectiveness of health-care delivery

In theory, and as demonstrated in the United States in practice,[12] private insurers can employ market power in the same way public health systems employ power as regulators or monopsonists to promote cost-effective health-care delivery. In part, this could entail use of tools for health-care management. The concept of "managed care" encompasses a variety of initiatives directed at influencing the quantity, quality, and appropriateness of care provided to insurees. These include, for example, health prevention and promotion initiatives, management of chronic conditions, utilisation review, clinical guidelines, restrictions on treatments, and incentives or information directed to consumers to promote choice of cost-effective providers or services. Also in part, insurers' initiatives to promote cost-effective health-care delivery could include selection of providers on the basis of cost-effectiveness considerations.

In most OECD countries, private insurers have not implemented measures to enhance the cost-effectiveness of the health-care services they finance. Several explanations for the limited involvement of insurers in managing care are plausible, including, among others, complexity and cost, resistance by the medical profession and desire not to restrict individual choice. Furthermore, in most OECD countries, insurers have not leveraged the potential of selective provider contracting to strengthen their ability to negotiate care-management arrangements with providers. Notably, many of these same considerations apply to public purchasers, as well. However, in a single-payer system, there is an additional factor in that it may be more difficult, from a policy-making perspective, for a publicly financed monopsonist to differentiate treatment of health-care providers.

Managed-care tools require sophistication to use, and organisations and insurers may have limited incentives to invest in their application, especially if they do not expect significant gains, or anticipate opposition by stakeholders such as professional associations. Incentives to manage care for high-risk and high-cost cases are also reduced by insurers' limited exposure to risk and cost in countries where private health insurance has a minor role in financing more costly care. Pooling arrangements that share the cost of care of vulnerable individuals (whether voluntary or mandatory) promote equitable risk sharing across insurers, but reduce their incentives to manage care efficiently.

While insurers in the United States have more actively sought to influence health-care delivery patterns, volumes and costs, some of these efforts raised access concerns and have been altered by a combination of voluntary market changes and increased regulation. In the United States, employers' efforts to reduce costs through the use of managed care is widely credited with efficiency improvements – such as declines in lengths of hospital stays – that slowed health-cost growth in the 1990s. These successes are largely attributable to selective contracting, which limited enrolees' choice of provider, combined with limitations in provider reimbursement levels, as well as utilisation controls. Resistance from providers and consumers led employers and individuals to demand more flexibility in their coverage arrangements (often referred to as the "backlash" against managed care), driving health plans to modify their practices, often through looser controls over choice of provider and access to care.[13] Such phenomena show some of the limits of private insurance markets' ability to promote improvements in the cost-efficiency of health-care delivery. At the same time, they demonstrate the ability of such markets to adapt to demand.

Competition among health insurers as a tool for increasing health system efficiency

Some countries with private health insurance or multiple social insurers have sought to create competitive insurance markets. Competition for insurees and profits is expected to drive efficiency improvements and to increase responsiveness to innovation and purchasers' preferences and demands.

The extent to which competition actually occurs in health insurance markets of OECD countries is limited, however (see Box 5.3). Switching across insurers is hindered by high transaction and informational costs, and is complicated in some countries by the lack of portability of cover and the absence of comparative information on insurers' performance. Incentives to switch insurance products are minimised where there is little differentiation of product or premium. The small size of the private health insurance markets, particularly where private insurance is not the main source of coverage for the population, may limit incentives for insurers to enter the market. For historical reasons, several private health insurance markets are dominated by a small number of insurers that may draw membership from given regions or employment groups.

Competition in health insurance markets, where it occurs, does not automatically deliver intended improvements in cost-efficiency. Much depends on the grounds on which insurers compete. Insurers operating in markets that appear to be more competitive face incentives to compete not only on the basis of real efficiency gains, but

> ### Box 5.3. **Experience with increasing competition among insurers in OECD countries**
>
> Reforms designed to promote competition among social and private insurers have been introduced in Belgium, Germany, the Netherlands, and Switzerland, building on the presence of multiple insurers. Insurance-market competition can improve efficiency in two ways. First, it encourages insurers to minimise administrative costs and improve their services to the insured (even though they are still likely to have higher administrative expenses when compared with countries with a single payer). Second, selective contracting by insurers among competing health-care suppliers – following the approach in managed-care markets in the United States – can encourage more efficient health-care provision.
>
> Recent experience in countries that have introduced competition suggests that it may be more difficult than anticipated to achieve and maintain competition under the constraint of maintaining full population coverage. Short-run experience suggests that competing social insurers have led to an evening-out of premiums between insurers but the extent of this is quite variable across countries.[1] The key question over the longer haul is whether this competition can be sustained, particularly given that with today's risk-adjustment techniques, insurers' incentives for "cream-skimming" cannot be fully eliminated. However, one important reason for having competing insurers is their potential ability to force providers to become more cost-efficient. Up to the present, regulations have limited such effects in most OECD countries: prices continue to be set in a bilateral monopoly environment and there is little oversight of providers by insurers regarding the pertinence and quality of care.
>
> Potential evidence on the benefits of insurance market competition has been provided by a comparison between Kaiser Permanente, the California health maintenance organisation and the British National Health Service (NHS) (Feachem et al., 2002). Both are integrated models of health care but Kaiser competes for insurees in the market with other plans whereas the NHS enjoys a monopoly of publicly funded health care for all UK citizens. A statistical comparison suggests that Kaiser achieved better performance at roughly the same cost as the NHS. The suggested reasons include: better integration across the system, better management of hospital resources and greater investment in information technology. This gives rise to the suggestion that an organisation challenged by competition will be forced to find ways to become more efficient than a monopoly, if it is to survive. On the other hand, Kaiser itself is having difficulty competing in US insurance markets, partly because its reputation for quality encourages enrolment by higher-risk people, resulting in adverse selection and higher premiums compared to other plans.
>
> 1. There has been some move of clients from high-cost to low-cost insurers and the extent has depended to some degree on the initial differences in the size of the premium between insurers. Thus, the movements of insured and the narrowing of premiums have been larger in Germany where the starting differences were larger than in the Netherlands where they were small. However, despite very large differences in premiums in Switzerland, there has been relatively little movement as individuals have strong local loyalty to existing insurers.

also through risk selection and other practices that shift costs to other payers. In Australia, for example, insurers can benefit from offering less comprehensive products that attract lower-risk individuals. Private insurers that provide optional duplicate coverage to beneficiaries of the US Medicare programme tend to attract lower risks, and beneficiaries who develop health problems may revert to the standard public coverage, raising public costs. From a technical and policy standpoint, it is very difficult to counter these incentives, which can be strong, given that a small share of the insured population accounts for a large share of health costs. Insurers also need to sustain high overhead costs linked to advertising, billing, product innovation and contracting with providers, adding to costs in competitive markets.

Adequate regulatory and informational tools are required to steer insurers towards efficiency-based competition, especially when equity considerations are paramount, as when private health insurance represents a primary form of cover for certain sections of the population or when it covers essential services. Regulatory safeguards are needed to enhance competition in a private health insurance market because of market imperfections such as information asymmetry and insurers' incentives to encourage enrolment and retention of lower-risk persons. Individuals need transparent information and consumer protection regulation to become confident in, and knowledgeable about, the products they are buying.

Approaches for increasing efficiency: summary of findings

Evidence points to significant inefficiency in OECD health systems that could be addressed through appropriate changes in policy. Notably, it is not clear whether countries have invested adequately in efforts to prevent disease and promote health. It appears likely that systems have devoted excessive resources to health care at the expense of prevention, a possibility that requires careful further exploration, although there is no assurance that the cost-effectiveness of any given investment in prevention will necessarily be greater than the cost-effectiveness of the subsequent cure.

Changes on the demand side offer some prospects. Especially in systems where health care is essentially free and unrestricted, from the perspective of the user of services, there may be room for improvement in the cost-effectiveness of health-care delivery by implementing some demand management, such as gatekeepers. In addition, approaches such as informing patients about the costs and expected outcomes for certain treatments, and using reference pricing for pharmaceutical drugs, stand to improve efficiency. Cost-sharing requirements might be employed in a more discriminating manner, freeing up funds for coverage expansions (populations or core benefits) in ways that could enhance efficiency. Private health insurance that complements public coverage by picking up patient cost-sharing requirements has a significant downside, in that it blunts patient price sensitivity, thereby limiting efforts to improve efficiency through such approaches as reference-pricing for pharmaceuticals. On the other hand, supplementary private insurance may be useful as a mechanism for rationing based on price for ancillary services, luxuries, or services judged by policy makers as non-essential.

On the supply side, there is perhaps more promise. Efforts to distinguish the roles of health-care payers and providers, more closely mirroring normal economic markets, have proved generally effective. There is potential for further organisational reforms, such as decentralisation or management changes, to reduce waste, increase productivity and enhance systems' cost-effectiveness. Efficient deployment of human resources may be enhanced by substituting lower-skilled workers, such as nurse practitioners for physicians, under appropriate circumstances.

Absent price rationing or demand management, demand for many services is likely to be higher than policy makers in some countries are willing to finance publicly. Therefore, some management of capacity and supply of services is likely to be appropriate in many systems so as to steer diffusion of new technology. This should be undertaken using the best information possible, as evaluated through technology assessment programmes, and employing mechanisms designed to promote cost-effective health-care delivery, rather than blunt approaches. Some minimal waiting times for elective surgery may be considered appropriate in some systems as an indicator that there is not excess surgical capacity in a system, although it is important to assess whether productivity shortfalls play a role. The extent to which maintaining waiting times is appropriate is entirely dependent on the value assigned to various marginal improvements in perceived responsiveness, patient quality of life and outcomes, as well as other social costs associated with waiting.

Policy makers face real challenges in promoting continued advances in medicine while managing communal resources appropriately. A free-rider problem exists, in that funding of research and development, as well as experience-based testing of the effects of innovation in health technology, occurs disproportionately in certain countries. Whether this approach is efficient and sustainable, or whether there is a better approach to this dilemma, is as yet unclear.

A key question is which approaches will create the best incentives for providers to increase the efficiency of health-care delivery. The experience with competition-based approaches has not, in general, been promising so far. Notable success with insurance-based competition in the US system was short-lived. Efforts in other countries, whether for private or social insurers, have been less successful. The extent to which competition versus payment incentives or other approaches are appropriate is likely to depend on whether there is excess supply in the system, the technical ability of purchasers to adopt sophisticated purchasing strategies, and other factors.

Across the OECD, payment methods for hospitals, physicians, and other health-care providers have evolved in a positive direction, a trend to be encouraged. Payments have moved away from cost-reimbursement, which favours inefficiency, towards an activity-based system. But systems that reward productivity have risks: risk of promoting service volume that is too high and of low marginal benefit. Far better would be payments that provide incentives to provide the right services at the right time, and that reward providers or organisations who contribute to system performance goals. Accomplishing such a change is fraught with challenges at both policy and technical levels. OECD countries are still a long way from this, but recent steps to move in this direction are a promising development that should be expanded.

The question of the interplay of long-term care with other health and social services should be seen as a question of whether cost control and efficiency of health and long-term care services can be improved through better cross-sector co-ordination. Ongoing efficiency gains in the hospital sector have increased the need for more readily accessible and more intensive long-term care services for older persons, in particular with the overall goal to prevent permanent institutionalisation after an episode of post-acute-care services. This and related interface issues will need further attention as cross-cutting issues between acute health care, long-term care (both health and social services) and other social services.

Notes

1. In addition to the structural or cross-cutting reforms discussed in this section of the report, supply-side initiatives focused on human resources for health care, the hospital sector, long-term care, technology management, and private health insurance are discussed in subsequent sections.

2. For example, research in the United States showed that moving to episode-based, prospective payment of hospitals by the public Medicare program in 1983 reduced length of stay, but did not hurt patient outcomes. More recently, changes undertaken by the US Veterans Health Administration resulted in a dramatic drop in hospital admissions, lengths of stay and emergency room use, while one-year survival rates for nine serious conditions improved or remained stable (Ashton et al., 2003).

3. Set too high, they provide rents to the hospital. Set too low, the hospital will not cover costs and may have to close.

4. For example, hospitals can have a fixed share of patients that are paid on a full-cost basis or have full reimbursement for patients with costs above a certain level.

5. This may have been the case in the Czech Republic in the early 1990s and in the ambulatory care sector in Germany in the second half of the 1990s.

6. The cost of bringing a new drug to market was recently as estimated at USD 880 million over 15 years (Tollman et al., 2001).

7. Italy and Sweden are amongst the countries that have introduced measures that award higher prices to products that demonstrate better cost-effectiveness, as compared to alternatives (Ekelund and Persson, 2003).

8. For example, in a systematic review of 33 interventions to treat acute and chronic lower back and neck pain, the Swedish Council of Health Technology Assessment (SBU) showed that in 44% of interventions, there was no evidence, and in a further 29%, there was only limited or moderate evidence. In 13% of interventions, there was evidence that the treatment was not effective (SBU, 2000).

9. For example, positron emission scanning was referenced in 19 708 articles between 1969 and 2002. The first health technology assessment appeared in 1979; since then, the technology has been assessed at least 454 times (OECD, 2004d).

10. The limited evidence on the impact of health technology assessment on decision-making is mixed. Two recent reports state that concrete examples of the impact of health technology assessment were hard to find and that the evidence base on how to translate evidence into practice is very limited (ECHTA, 2002; Maynard et al., 2000). In part, this result is a reflection of the complexity of measuring impact. However, a number of studies have examined the broader impact of health technology assessment. For example, Jacob and McGregor (1997) examined impact on policy decisions. They measured the impact that 16 health technology assessment reports had on the number of relevant regulations proposed, passed and enforced, and found that 12 of the reports had had considerable impact.

11. For example, one study found a lower rate of MRI use in areas with higher managed-care penetration (Baker and Wheeler, 1998). But another showed comparable rates of diffusion of advanced gallbladder surgery care between managed-care and traditional insurance plans (Chernew et al., 1997).

12. A few insurers in the United Kingdom have also put in place some limited quality-related efforts.

13. The issue is complicated by the US tax treatment of health insurance benefits, which encourages employer provision and minimises the extent to which employees are sensitive to the costs of insurance policies.

ISBN 92-64-01555-8
Towards High-Performing Health Systems
© OECD 2004

Conclusions from the OECD Health Project: promising approaches for improving health-system performance

The pay-off from years of experimentation and investigation is that health policy makers in OECD countries now know quite a bit about which tools and approaches can be used successfully to accomplish many key policy objectives, such as controlling the rate of public spending growth, ensuring equitable access to care, improving health and preventing disease, and establishing equitable and sustainable financing for health and long-term care services. Recent OECD work has added to the tool kits, offering valuable lessons relevant to many of the most pressing policy concerns on the effects of various policies intended to manage the adoption and diffusion of health-related technology, address shortages of nurses and other health-care workers, increase the productivity of hospitals and physicians, manage the demand for health services, reduce waiting times for elective surgery, and foster the availability of affordable private health insurance coverage (see Box). In addition, further light has been shed on dilemmas such as judging the appropriate level of health spending, assessing the appropriate role for private financing in health and long-term care systems and evaluating the implications of waiting times for elective surgery.

Despite the plethora of information and experience-based guidance available, attaining health-system performance goals has proven to be a far from simple task. Health is an area of the economy that has experienced considerable government intervention based on public interest, some of which undoubtedly result in regulatory failures and distortions, and also suffers from serious market failures when government interventions are minimal. Nevertheless, there is no doubt that countries have improved the performance of their health systems over time and made big advances towards key policy goals. Failure to meet fully many outstanding goals partly reflects the important effect of institutional and historical context on the outcome of various approaches to improvement. Certainly, it also reflects implementation challenges that influence the ability to make changes in line with intentions. In the health sector as in other areas of policy making, there are always stakeholders who benefit from the status quo and will oppose changes perceived as a threat to their self-interest. Reconciling social and industrial goals can be particularly challenging in the health sector. But perhaps most importantly, outstanding policy challenges reflect the interdependence of various dimensions of performance, so as to make trade-offs between them, intended and unintended, almost impossible to avoid. Because policy makers will place different values on different goals, there is no one-size-fits-all approach to best policy-making in the health sector.

Health policy-making involves a careful balance of trade-offs, reflecting the weights assigned to a range of important goals and a great deal of uncertainty regarding both intended and unintended consequences of various decisions. The ultimate goal, certainly, is robust population health, but promoting health is often not the only objective taken into account in making health policy decisions. The health sector is a strong and important component of the economies of OECD member countries, providing extensive employment and profitable industry, and making the economic consequences

Promising directions for health policy

Findings from the OECD Health Project point to a number of useful practices or approaches that can be employed in efforts to improve health-system performance. As these typically imply trade-offs with competing policy goals, policy makers must determine whether the expected benefits from these practices are likely to outweigh the costs in a particular situation. In addition, a country's unique circumstances must be taken into account when determining appropriate policy. There is no one-size-fits-all approach to performance improvement.

Possible lines of action for improving population health status and health outcomes

● Employ well-designed strategies to prevent illness and disability, which may entail reallocations of health-system resources from care to prevention, or changes in the way resources are spent. Evaluate the potential to improve health through changes in policy (including taxation) relating to nutrition, violence, traffic, alcohol or tobacco use, or other areas that may fall outside the strict purview of health policy-making.

● Address inequities in health through initiatives targeted at tackling root causes, such as poverty and social exclusion, in addition to ones targeted at improving health care for vulnerable populations.

● Support efforts to increase the extent to which medical practice is consistent with evidence – including development and implementation of evidence-based practice guidelines and performance standards, and alignment of economic and administrative incentives with use of appropriate care and attainment of desired health outcomes.

● Ensure that systems for monitoring the quality of health and long-term care are sufficient to assist in meeting improvement goals. Development and standardisation of valid quality indicators, including measures of health outcomes, are essential steps.

Possible lines of action for fostering adequate and equitable access to care

● Eliminate financial barriers to access by providing or subsidising health coverage for the poor, exempting poor persons from patient cost-sharing requirements, and allowing complementary private health insurance to cover a portion of user fees in cases where these are high enough to create access barriers.

● Foster access to affordable private health insurance by high-risk persons (*e.g.* the elderly and those with costly medical conditions), where such coverage is needed to assure access to care, through interventions such as targeted regulations, subsidies or fiscal incentives.

● Avoid unintended inequities in access by persons with different sources of health coverage through policy interventions such as universally applicable provider reimbursement limits or employment of common waiting lists.

Possible lines of action for increasing health-system responsiveness

● Reduce waiting times for elective surgery, where they are judged to be excessive, by increasing surgical capacity or productivity (through a change in provider payment methods, for example).

● Improve recipient satisfaction with long-term care by supporting family caregivers and/ or, so as to increase care recipients' control over services and choice of providers, offering cash payments for spending on services directly to those eligible for benefits.

● Facilitate informed consumer choice of health insurance coverage, whether publicly or privately financed.

Promising directions for health policy *(cont.)*

Possible lines of action for ensuring sustainable costs and financing

- Moderate the rate of growth in public spending on health through a combination of budgetary and administrative controls over payments, prices or supply of services. Monitor carefully the effects of such interventions on health-system performance.

- Add modest cost-sharing requirements to publicly financed health coverage schemes and bar complementary health insurance from covering, in full, the amount to be paid by the patient.

- Eliminate public coverage for ancillary or luxury services, allowing for rationing by price and optional risk-pooling through privately financed supplementary coverage.

Possible lines of action for increasing the efficiency of health systems

- Manage demand for elective surgery and other discretionary care through gatekeepers, clinical prioritisation, or consumer and patient information schemes, particularly in systems where low patient cost-sharing and excess supply of health-care providers combine to promote high levels of service use.

- Employ pharmaceutical pricing systems and other policies that reward cost-effective choices among similar medications and encourage truly novel innovation in the pharmaceutical sector.

- Use technology assessment to promote informed decision-making, and use technology-management approaches that take health outcomes into account and promote cost-effective health-care delivery.

- Develop, test and employ payment systems for health-care services that reward productivity and quality.

Possible lines of action for improving overall health-system performance

- Invest in automated health-data systems needed to improve the organisation and delivery of health care.

- Monitor health-system performance regularly, using valid indicators and reliable data, and benchmark against established goals or the performance of peers (through international comparisons).

of health policy decisions considerable. Social and political considerations are important, as well, in that the extent to which health systems and health care satisfy patients, consumers, and other stakeholders is seen as a critical factor in health-system performance. Also important is the fact that it is very difficult to disentangle the effects of health systems on health status, given that a variety of socio-economic factors, as well as behavioural and risk factors, also play an important role.

Health systems differ widely in their design, in the inputs they employ and the outcomes they attain. Yet OECD countries have endorsed a very similar set of performance goals and virtually all face a common objective of improving the performance of their health systems. In terms of improving the performance of health systems in meeting the goals policy makers set for them, the path ahead is clear: OECD countries can only benefit from further experimentation, combined with conscientious performance measurement using actionable and specific indicators, benchmarking, and sharing of information on approaches taken, experiences and outcomes, so as to uncover effective and ineffective practices and the circumstances under which various approaches can work.

Improving health system performance will require changes to health systems. This is likely to require some up-front investments that will be cost-effective, if not cost saving, in the long run. At the very least, improvements will require better systems for recording, storing, accessing, and transferring health data, and for monitoring and assessing performance (OECD, 2002). Realigning economic incentives of health-care providers, patients, and health-care organisations is also in order, and health-care purchasers (both public and private) need to become more sophisticated in their efforts to attain value for money. Health systems, providers and organisations that have some financial margin for operating may be better positioned to make needed investments that allow for improvements in the cost-effectiveness of health-care delivery, but even cash-strapped systems may be able find ways to reduce waste and increase productivity if given incentives to do so. Health care is a rapidly evolving field. The organisation of health care needs to evolve along with it. Systems can benefit from flexibility and an ability to change and evolve with new evidence.

While recent work at the OECD has filled a number of knowledge gaps, numerous important policy questions are outstanding, many of which were uncovered in the course of this work. Among the most urgent issues, given today's goals, are the following: How can competitive market forces be better employed to increase the efficiency of health systems? How can continued advances in medical technology be promoted and timely access to new developments be assured while managing public resources responsibly? In light of both market and regulatory failures, which approaches work best to ensure an adequate future supply of health workers? How can the economic incentives of health-care providers be better aligned with goals for cost-effective health-care delivery? Which approaches to medical professional liability can best deter negligence, compensate victims, encourage appropriate use of health services, and allow for learning from mistakes for future quality improvement? Further work at an international level can assist policy makers in formulating evidence-based answers to these questions.

ISBN 92-64-01555-8
Towards High-Performing Health Systems
© OECD 2004

Bibliography

Aaron, H. (2003), "Should Public Policy Seek to Control the Growth of Health Care Spending?", *Health Affairs*, January.

Agency for Healthcare Research and Quality (2000), "Medical Errors: The Scope of the Problem", Fact sheet, Publication No. AHRQ 00-P037, Rockville, MD. Available at *www.ahrq.gov/qual/errback.htm*.

Agency for Healthcare Research and Quality (2001), "Reducing and Preventing Adverse Drug Events to Decrease Hospital Costs. Research in Action", Issue 1: AHRQ Publication Number 01-0020, March, Rockville, MD. Available at *www.ahrq.gov/qual/aderia/aderia.htm*.

Aiken, L.H., Clarke, S.P., Cheung, R.B., Sloane, D.M. and Silber, J.H. (2003), "Educational Levels of Hospital Nurses and Surgical Patient Mortality", *Journal of the American Medical Association*, Vol. 290, No. 12, pp. 1617-1623.

Alter, D.A., Iron, K., Austin, P. and Naylor, D. (2004), "Socioeconomic Status, Service Patterns, and Perceptions of Care Among Survivors of Acute Myocardial Infarction in Canada", *JAMA*, Vol. 291, No. 9, pp. 1100-1107.

Alter, D.A., Naylor, C.D., Austin, P. and Tu, J.V. (1999), "Effects of Socioeconomic Status on Access to Invasive Cardiac Procedures and on Mortality after Acute Myocardial Infarction", *New England Journal of Medicine*, Vol. 341, pp. 1359-1367.

Antonazzo, E., Scott, A., Skatun, D. and Elliott, R.F. (2003), "The Labour Market for Nursing: A Review of the Labour Supply Literature", *Health Economics*, Vol. 12, pp. 465-478.

Ashton, C.M., Souchek, J., Petersen, N.J., Menke, T.J., Collins, T.C., Kizer, K.W., Wright, S.M. and Wray, N.P. (2003), "Hospital Use and Survival Among Veterans Affairs Beneficiaries",*New England Journal of Medicine*, Oct. 23, Vol. 349(17), pp. 1637-1646.

Bains, M. and Oxley, H. (2004), "Ageing-related Spending Projections for Health and Long-term Care", *Towards Higher-Performing Health Systems: Policy Studies from the OECD Health Project*, forthcoming.

Baker, L.C. and Wheeler, S.K. (1998), "Managed Care and Technology Diffusion: the Case of MRI", *Health Affairs*, Vol. 17(5), Sept.-Oct., pp. 195-207.

Beasley, R., Pearce, N. and Crane, J. (1997), "International Trends in Asthma Mortality", *Ciba Found Symposium*, Discussion 150-6 and 157-9, Vol. 206, pp. 140-150.

Bennett, J. (2003), "Investment in Population Health in Five OECD Countries", OECD Health Working Papers, No. 2, OECD, Paris.

Bernstein, S.J., Brorsson, B., Aberg, T., Emanuelsson, H., Brook, R.H. and Werko, L. (1999), "Appropriateness of Referral of Coronary Angiography Patients in Sweden. SECOR/SBU Project Group", *Heart*, Vol. 81, No. 5, pp. 470-477, May.

Birmingham, C.L. *et al.* (1999), "The Cost of Obesity in Canada", *Canadian Medical Association Journal*, Vol. 160, No. 4, pp. 483-488, February 23.

Bishai, D.M. and Lang, H.C. (2000), "The Willingness to Pay for Wait Reduction: the Disutility of Queues for Cataract Surgery in Canada, Denmark and Spain", *Journal of Health Economics*, Vol. 19, pp. 219-230.

Blendon, R.J., Schoen, C., Desroches, C.M., Osborn, R., Scoles, K.L. and Zapert, K. (2002), "Inequities in Health Care: a Five-Country Survey", *Health Affairs*, Vol. 21(3), pp. 182-190, May/June.

Bowker, T.J., Clayton, T.C., Ingham, J. *et al.* (1996), "A British Cardiac Society Survey of the Potential for the Secondary Prevention of Coronary Disease: ASPIRE (Action on Secondary Prevention through Intervention to Reduce Events)", *Heart*, Vol. 75, pp. 334-342.

Canadian Institute for Health Information (2003), *Drug Expenditure in Canada, 1985 to 2002*, Canadian Institute for Health Information, Canada.

Chassin, M.R. and Galvin, R.W. (1998), "The Urgent Need to Improve Health Care Quality", Institute of Medicine National Roundtable on Health Care Quality, *JAMA*, Vol. 280, pp. 1000–1005.

Chernew, M., Fendrick, A.M. and Hirth, R.A. (1997), "Managed Care and Medical Technology: Implications for Cost Growth", *Health Affairs*, Mar.-Apr., Vol. 16(2), pp. 196-206.

Colombo, F. (2001), "Towards More Choice in Social Protection? Individual Choice of Insurer in Basic Mandatory Health Insurance in Switzerland", Labour Market and Social Policy Occasional Papers, No. 53, OECD, Paris.

Cowan, D. and Turner-Smith, A. (1998), "The Role of Assistive Technology in Alternative Models of Care for Elderly People", Appendix 4 in A. Tinker., F. Wright, C. McCreadie, J. Askham, R. Hancock and A. Holmans (eds.) (1999), *Alternative Models of Care for Older People (With Respect to Old Age: Long-Term Care – Rights and Responsibilities: A Report by the Royal Commission on Long-Term Care)*, Research Volume 2, The Stationary Office, London. *www.archive.official-documents.co.uk/document/cm41/4194/4192-2v2.htm* (accessed December 2003).

Cox, J.L. *et al.* (1996), "Managed Delay for Coronary Artery Bypass Graft Surgery: the Experience at One Canadian Center", *Journal of the American College of Cardiology*, Vol. 27, pp. 1365-1373.

Cutler, D. and McClellan, M. (2001), "Is Technological Change in Medicine Worth It?", *Health Affairs*, Vol. 20, No. 5, Sept./Oct.

Dang, T.T., Antolin, P. and Oxley, H. (2001), "Fiscal Implications of Ageing: projections of age-related spending", OECD Economic Department Working Papers, No. 305, OECD, Paris.

Davies, B. and Fernandez, J.L. (2003), "Evaluating Community Care for Elderly People", *PSSRU Bulletin 14*, Personal Social Services Research Unit, University of Kent, Canterbury, UK.

Dickson, M. *et al.* (2003), "Survey of Pharmacoeconomic Assessment Activity in Eleven Countries", OECD Health Working Papers, No. 4, OECD, Paris.

Docteur, E. and Oxley, H. (2003), "Health Care Systems: Lessons from the Reform Experience", OECD Economics Department Working Papers, No. 374 and Health Working Papers, No. 9, OECD, Paris.

Docteur, E., Suppanz, H. and Woo, J. (2003), "The US Health System: an assessment and prospective directions for reform", OECD Economics Department Working Paper, No. 350, OECD, Paris.

Domberger, S. and Jensen, P. (1997), "Contracting out by the Public Sector: theory, evidence and prospects", *Oxford Review of Economic Policy*, Vol. 13, No. 4, pp. 67-78.

Doody, R.S., Stevens, J.C., Beck, C., Dubinsky, R.M., Kaye, J.A., Gwyther, L., Mohs, R.C., Thal, L.J., Whitehouse, P.J., Dekosky, S.T. and Cummings, J.L. (2001), "Practice Parameter: Management of Dementia (an Evidence-based Review): Report of the Quality Standards Subcommittee of the American Academy of Neurology", *Neurology*, May 8, Vol. 56(9), pp. 1154-1166.

Doolan, D.F. and Bates, D.W. (2002), "Computerized Physician Order Entry Systems in Hospitals: Mandates and Incentives", *Health Affairs*, Vol. 21(4), July/August, pp. 180-188.

DREES – Direction de la recherche, des études, de l'évaluation et des statistiques (2003), "L'impact de la CMU sur la consommation individuelle de soins", *Études et résultats*, No. 229, March.

Duran, L. and Coburn, D. (2003), "The Use of Health Care Technology Information in the Health System Decision-Making Process", Draft working paper produced for The OECD's New and Emerging Health-Related Technology Project.

ECHTA – European Collaboration for Health Technology Assessment Project (2002), "Working Group 6 Report", *International Journal of Health Technology Assessment in Health Care*, Vol. 18, No. 2, pp. 447-455.

Ekelund, M. and Persson, B. (2003), "Pharmaceutical Pricing in a Regulated Market", *Review of Economics and Statistics*, Vol. 85(2), pp. 298-306.

EuroAspire I and II Group (2001), "Clinical Reality of Coronary Prevention Guidelines: A Comparison of EuroAspire I and II in Nine Countries", *Lancet*, Vol. 357, pp. 995-1001.

European Commission (2001), *Key Figures on Health Pocketbook*.

Feachem, R.G. *et al.* (2002), "Getting More for their Dollar: A Comparison of the NHS with California's Kaiser Permanente", *British Medical Journal*, Vol. 324, pp. 135-142.

Fonds de Financement de la CMU (2003), *Rapport d'évaluation de la CMU*, Paris, December.

Forsberg, E., Axelsson, R. and Arnetz, B. (2001), "Financial Incentives in Health Care. The Impact of Performance-based Reimbursement", *Health Affairs*, Vol. 58.

Frost and Sullivan (2001), *US Tissue Engineering Market*, 26 September.

Fuchs, V.R. (1987), "The Counterrevolution in Health Care Financing", *New England Journal of Medicine* Vol. 316(18), pp. 1154-1156.

Gelijns, A. *et al.* (2004), "The Potential and Pitfalls of Evidence-based Decision-making for Technology: Issues in Transferability", Draft working paper produced for The OECD's New and Emerging Health-Related Technology Project.

Gosden T., Pederson, L. and Torgerson, D. (1999), "How Should we Pay Doctors? A Systematic Review of Salary Payments and their Effect on Doctor Behaviour", *Quarterly Journal of Medicine*, Vol. 92, pp. 47-55.

Gosden, T., Forland, F., Kristiansen, I.S., Sutton, M., Leese, B., Giuffrida, A., Sergison, M. and Pedersen, L. (2001), "Impact of Payment Method on Behaviour of Primary Care Physicians: A Systematic Review", *Journal of Health Services Research and Policy*, Vol. 6, No. 1, pp. 44-55.

Gray, D., Hampton, J.R., Bernstein, S.J., Kosecoff, J., Brook, R.H. (1990), "Audit of Coronary Angiography and Bypass Surgery", *Lancet*, Vol. 335(8701), pp. 1317-1320, June 2.

Gress, S., Groenewegen, P., Kerssens, J., Braun, B. and Wasem, J. (2002), "Free Choice of Sickness Fund in Regulated Competition: Evidence from Germany and the Netherlands", *Health Policy*, No. 60, No. 3, pp. 235-254, June.

Hadley, J. (2002), *Sicker and Poorer: The Consequences of Being Uninsured*, Kaiser Family Foundation, May.

Halm, E.A. and Gelijns, A.C. (1991), "An Introduction to the Changing Economics of Technical Innovation in Medicine", in A.C. Gelijns and E.A. Halm (eds.), *The Changing Economics of Medical Technology*, National Academy Press, Washington DC.

Halm, E.A., Chassin, M.R., Tuhrim, S., Hollier, L.H., Popp, A.J., Ascher, E., Dardik, H., Faust, G. and Riles, T.S. (2003), "Revisiting the Appropriateness of Carotid Endarterectomy", *Stroke*, Vol. 34(6), pp. 1464-1471, June.

Hawes, C., Phillips, C.D., Rose, M., Holan, S. and Sherman, M. (2003), "A National Survey of Assisted Living Facilities", *The Gerontologist*, Vol. 43, pp. 875-882.

Heidenreich, P.A. and McClellan, M. (2001), "Trends in Treatment and Outcomes for Acute Myocardial Infarction: 1975-1995", *American Journal of Medicine*, Vol. 110(3), pp. 165-174, February 15.

Hetemaa, I., Keskimäki, I., Manderbacka, K., Leyland, A.H. and Koskinen, S. (2003), "How Did the Recent Increase in the Supply of Coronary Operations in Finland Affect Socio-economic and Gender Inequity in their Use?", *Journal of Epidemiology and Community Health*, Vol. 57, pp. 178-185.

Hill, S., Garattini, S., Van Loenhout, J., O'Brien, B.J. and DeJoncheere, K. (2003), *Technology Appraisal Programme of the National Institute for Clinical Excellence – A Review by WHO*, World Health Organization – Europe.

Himmelstein, D.U. and Woolhandler, S. (1986), "Cost without Benefit. Administrative Waste in US Health Care", *New England Journal of Medicine*, Vol. 314(7), pp. 441-445, February.

Hirose, M., Imanacka, Y., Tasuro, I. and Evans, E. (2003), "How Can We Improve the Quality of Health Care in Japan? Learning from JCQHC Hospital Accreditation", *Health Policy*, Vol. 66, pp. 29-49.

Hisashige, A. (1992), "The Introduction and Evaluation of MRI in Japan", *International Society for Technology Assessment in Health Care*, Vol. 3, No. 126.

Hollander, M. and Chappell, N. (2002), *Final Report of the National Evaluation of the Cost-effectiveness of Home Care: A Report Prepared for the Health Transition Fund, Health Canada*, National Evaluation of the Cost-Effectiveness of Home Care, Victoria, British Columbia.

Hughes, M. (2003), "Summary of Results from Breast Cancer Disease Study," *A Disease-based Comparison of Health Systems: What is Best and at What Cost?*, OECD, Paris.

Hunt, L.W., Silverstein, M.D., Reed, C.E., O'Connell, E.J., O'Fallon, W.M. and Yunginger, J.W. (1993), "Accuracy of the Death Certificate in a Population-based Study of Asthmatic Patients", *JAMA*, Vol. 269(15), pp. 1947-1952.

Hurst, J. and Siciliani, L. (2003), "Tackling Excessive Waiting Times for Elective Surgery: A Comparison of Policies in Twelve OECD Countries", OECD Health Working Papers, No. 6, OECD, Paris.

Institute of Medicine (1991), *The Computer-based Patient Record: An Essential Technology for Health Care*, in R.S. Dick and E.B. Steen (eds.),National Academy Press, Washington DC.

Institute of Medicine (1999), *To Err is Human: Building a Safer Health System*, in L.T. Kohn, J.M. Corrigan and M.S. Donaldson (eds.), National Academy Press, Washington DC.

Institute of Medicine (2001), *Crossing the Quality Chasm: A New Health System for the 21st Century* National Academy Press, Washington DC.

Jacob, R. and McGregor, M. (1997), "Assessing the Impact of Health Technology Assessment", *International Journal of Technology Assessment in Health Care*, Vol. 13, pp. 68-80.

Jacobzone, S., Cambois, E., Chaplain, E. and Robine, J.M. (1998), "The Health of Older Persons in OECD Countries: Is it Improving Fast Enough to Compensate for Population Ageing?", Labour Market and Social Policy Occasional Papers, No. 37, OECD, Paris.

Jencks, S.F., Huff, E.D. and Cuerdon, T. (2003), "Change in the Quality of Care Delivered to Medicare Beneficiaries, 1998-1999 to 2000-2001", *Journal of the American Medical Association*, Vol. 289, pp. 305-312.

Jencks, S.F., Cuerdon, T., Burwen, D.R., Fleming, B., Houck, P.M., Kussmaul, A.E., Nilasena, D.S., Ordin, D.L. and Arday, D.R. (2000), "Quality of Medical Care Delivered to Medicare Beneficiaries: A Profile at State and National Levels", *Journal of the American Medical Association*, Vol. 284, pp. 1670-1676.

Kalisch, D.W., Aaman, T. and Buchele, L.A. (1998), "Social and Health Policies in OECD Countries: A Survey of Current Programmes and Recent Developments", Labour Market and Social Policy Occasional Papers, No. 33, OECD, Paris.

Kamien, M. (1998), "Staying in or Leaving Rural Practice: 1996 Outcomes of Rural Doctors'1986 Intentions", *Medical Journal of Australia*, Vol. 169, pp. 318-321.

Katz, S.J., McMahon, L.F. and Manning, W.G. (1996), "Comparing the Use of Diagnostic Tests in Canadian and US Hospitals", *Medical Care*, Vol. 34, No. 2, pp. 117-125.

Keskimäki, I. (2003), "How Did Finland's Recession in the Early 1990s Affect Socio-economic Equity in the Use of Hospital Care?", *Social Science and Medicine*, Vol. 56, pp. 1517-1530.

Khuri, S.F., Daley, J., Henderson, W., Hur, K., Demakis, J., Aust, J.B., Chong, V., Fabri, P.J., Gibbs, J.O., Grover, F., Hammermeister, K., Irvin, G., McDonald, G., Passaro, E., Phillips, L., Scamman, F., Spencer, J. and Stremple, J.F. (1998), "The Department of Veterans Affairs' NSQIP: the first national, validated, outcome-based, risk-adjusted, and peer-controlled program for the measurement and enhancement of the quality of surgical care. National VA Surgical Quality Improvement Program", *Annals of Surgery*, Vol. 228(4), pp. 491-507.

Kili, S. *et al.* (2003), "Change in Harris Hip Score in Patients on the Waiting List for Total Hip Replacement", *Ann R. Coll. Sing. Engl.*, Vol. 85, pp. 269-271.

Kizer, K.W. (2000), "Reengineering the Veterans Healthcare System", in Ramsaroop *et al.* (eds.), *Advancing Federal Healthcare*, Spinger, New York.

Lafer, G., Moss, H., Kirtner, R. and Reese, V. (2003), *Solving the Nnursing Shortage. Best and Worst Practices for Recruiting, Retaining and Recouping of Hospital Nurses*, Labor Education and Research Center, University of Oregon.

Lanes, S.F., Birmann, B., Raiford, D. and Walker, A.M. (1997), "International Trends in Sales of Inhaled Fenoterol, All Inhaled Beta-agonists, and Asthma Mortality, 1970-1992", *Journal of Clinical Epidemiology*, Vol. 50(3), pp. 321-328, March.

Leape, L.L. (1994), "Error in Medicine", *Journal of the American Medical Association*, Vol. 272, pp. 1851-1857.

Lundsgaard, J. (2004), "Consumer Direction and Choice in Long-term Care for Older Persons", OECD Health Working Papers, OECD, Paris, forthcoming.

Manning, W.J. *et al.* (1987), "Health Insurance and the Demand for Medical Care: evidence from a randomised experiment", *American Economic Review*, Vol. 773 (June).

Mattke, S. (2004), "Monitoring and Improving the Technical Quality of Health Care", *Towards High-Performing Health Systems: Policy Studies from the OECD Health Project*, OECD, Paris, forthcoming.

Maynard, A. and Walker, A. (1997), *The Physician Workforce in the United Kingdom: Issues, Prospects and Policies*, The Nuffield Trust, Leeds.

Maynard, A., McDaid, D. and Astec (2000), "The Implications for Policy Makers", in R. Cookson, A. Maynard, D. McDaid, F. Sassi and T. Sheldon (eds.), *Analysis of the Scientific and Technical Evaluation of Health Care Interventions in the European Union. Report to European Commission*, July 2000. Available at *www.lse.ac.uk/Depts/lsehsc/astec_report.htm*

McClellan, M.B. and Kessler, D.P. (2003), "Conclusion", *Technological Change in Health Care: A Global Analysis of Heart Attack*, University of Michigan Press, Ann Arbor.

Medicare Payment Advisory Commission (2002), *Report to the Congress: Assessing Medicare Benefits*, Washington DC, June.

Moïse, P. (2003), "The Heart of the Health Care System: Summary of the Ischaemic Heart Disease Part of the OECD Ageing-related Diseases Study", *A Disease-based Comparison of Health Systems: What is Best and at What Cost?*, OECD, Paris.

Moïse, P., Schwarziner, M. and Um, M.Y. (2004), "The Future of Dementia and Alzheimer's Disease in OECD countries", OECD Health Working Papers, OECD, Paris, forthcoming.

Møldrup, C., Morgall, J.M. and Peck, J. (2003), "Methodological Developments in Medical Technology Assessment – The Prospective Approach", *International Journal of Risk Research*, Vol. 6, pp. 95-112.

Moon, L. (2003a), "Progressing the Collection of Information on Health Outcomes: A Perspective from the Ageing-related Diseases Study", *A Disease-based Comparison of Health Systems: What is Best and at What Cost?*, OECD, Paris.

Moon, L. (2003b), "Stroke Treatment and Care: A Comparison of Approaches in OECD Countries", *A Disease-based Comparison of Health Systems: What is Best and at What Cost?*, OECD, Paris.

NCQA – National Committee for Quality Assurance (2003), *The State of Health Care Quality: Industry Trends and Analysis*, NCQA, Washington, available at: *www.ncqa.org/Communications/ State%20Of%20Managed%20Care/SOHCREPORT2003.pdf*.

Newhouse, J.P. (1992), "Medical Care Costs: How Much Welfare Loss?", *Journal of Economic Perspectives*, Vol. 6, No. 3, Summer.

Newhouse, J.P. (2002), "Why is There a Quality Chasm?", *Health Affairs*, Vol. 21, pp. 13-25.

Nilsdotter, A.K. and Lohmander, L.S. (2002), "Age and Waiting Time as Predictors of Outcome after Total Hip Replacement for Osteoarthritis", *British Society for Rheumatology*, Vol. 41, pp. 1261-1266.

Nolte, E. and McKee, M. (2003), "Measuring the Health of Nations: Analysis of Mortality Amenable to Health Care", *BMJ*, Vol. 327, 15 November.

OECD (2001), *Ageing and Income, Financial Resources and Retirement in Nine OECD Countries*, Paris.

OECD (2002), *Measuring Up: Improving Health System Performance in OECD Countries*, Paris.

OECD (2003a), *Ageing, Housing and Urban Development*, Paris.

OECD (2003b), *A Disease-based Comparison of Health Systems: What is Best and at What Cost?*, Paris.

OECD (2003c), *Health at a Glance*, Paris.

OECD (2003d), *OECD Health Data, third edition*, Paris.

OECD (2003e), *OECD Reviews of Health Care Systems: Korea*, Paris.

OECD (2003f), *Trends in International Migration*, special chapter "The International Mobility of Health Profesionals: An Evaluation and Analysis Based on the Case of South Africa", Paris.

OECD (2004a), "Digital Delivery in Health Care", Chapter 5 in *Information Technology Outlook 2004*, Paris, forthcoming.

OECD (2004b), *Long-term Care for Older People*, OECD, Paris, forthcoming.

OECD (2004c), *Private Health Insurance in OECD Countries*, OECD, Paris, forthcoming.

OECD (2004d), *Health Technology and Decision Making*, OECD, Paris, forthcoming.

Pamolli, F. and Riccaboni, M. (2004), "Market Structure And Drug Innovation", *Health Affairs*, Vol. 23(1), pp. 48-50.

Partnership for Solutions (2002), *Chronic Conditions: Making the Case for Ongoing Care*, Baltimore, December, available at *www.partnershipforsolutions.org/DMS/files/chronicbook2002.pdf*.

Pritchard, C. (2002), "The Social and Economic Impact of Emerging Health Technologies: Mechanisms for Diffusion/Uptake of Technology and Evidence-based Planning", Document OECD DSTI(2002)1/ ANN1, OECD, Paris.

Propper, C. (1990), "Contingent Valuation of Time Spent on NHS Waiting Lists", *The Economic Journal*, Vol. 100 (Conference), pp. 193-199.

Propper, C. (1995), "The Disutility of Time Spent on the United Kingdom's National Health Service Waiting Lists", *The Journal of Human Resources*, pp. 677-700.

Rabinowitz, H.K., Diamond, J.J., Hojat, M. and Hazelwood, C.E. (1999), "Demographic, Educational and Economic Factors Related to Recruitment and Retention of Physicians in Rural Pennsylvania", *Journal of Rural Health*, Vol. 15, No. 2, pp. 212-218.

Reilly, T., Meyer, G., Zema, C., Crofton, C., Larson, D., Darby, C. and Crosson, K. (2002), "Providing Performance Information for Consumers: Experience from the United States", Chapter 5 in *Measuring Up: Improving Health System Performance in OECD Countries*, OECD, Paris.

Roos, L.L., Fisher, E.S., Brazauskas, R., Sharp, S.M. and Shapiro, E. (1992), "Health and Surgical Outcomes in Canada and the United States", *Health Affairs*, Vol. 11(2), pp. 56-72, Summer.

Roos, L.L., Fischer, E.S., Sharp, S.M., Newhouse, J.P., Anderson, G. and Bubolz, T.A. (1990), "Postsurgical Mortality in Manitoba and New England", *Journal of the American Medical Association*, Vol. 263(18), pp. 2453-2458.

Sarin, S. *et al.* (1993), "Does Venous Function Deteriorate in Patients Waiting for Varicose Vein Surgery?", *Journal of the Royal Society of Medicine*, Vol. 86, pp. 21-23.

SBU – Swedish Council of Technology Assessment in Health Care (2000), *Back Pain Neck Pain – An Evidence-based Review*, Report No. 145.

Schiøler, T., Lipczak, H., Pedersen, B.L., Torben, S., Mogensen, K., Bech, B.K., Stockmarr, A.A., Svenning, A.R. and Frolich, A. (2001), "Incidence of Adverse Events in Hospitalized Patients: The Danish Adverse Event Study (DAES)", *Ugeskr Læger*, Vol. 163, pp. 5370-5378.

Schneider, E.C., Zaslavsky, A.M. and Epstein, A.M. (2002), "Racial Disparities in the Quality of Care for Eenrollees in Medicare Managed Care", *Journal of the American Medical Association*, March 13, Vol. 287(10), pp. 1288-1294.

Shields, M.A. (2003), *The Global Shortage of Registered Nurses: What Can Policy-makers Learn from the Econometric Evidence on Nurse Labour Supply?*, Report Prepared for the Victorian Department of Treasury and Finance, Melbourne.

Siciliani, L. and Hurst, J. (2003), "Explaining Waiting Times Variations for Elective Surgery across OECD Countries", OECD Health Working Papers, No. 7, OECD, Paris.

Simoens, S. and Hurst, J. (2004), "Matching Supply and Demand for the Services of Physicians and Nurses", *Towards High-Performing Health Systems: Policy Studies*, OECD, Paris, forthcoming.

Siu, A.L., Sonnenberg, F. *et al.* (1986), "Inappropriate Use of Hospitals in a Randomized Trial of Health Insurance Plans", *New England Journal of Medicine*, Vol. 315, pp. 1259-1266.

Sturm, R. (2002), "The Effects of Obesity, Smoking, and Drinking on Medical Problems and Costs", *Health Affairs*, Vol. 21, No. 2, pp. 245-253, March/April.

Technological Change in Health Care (TECH) Research Network (2001), "Technological Change Around the World: Evidence from Heart Attack Care", *Health Affairs*, Vol. 20, No. 3, May/June.

Tinker, A. (2003), "Assistive Technology and its Role in Housing Policies for Older People", *Quality in Ageing – Policy, Practice and Research*, Vol. 4(2), pp. 4-12.

Tinker, A., Wright, F., McCreadie, C., Askham, J., Hancock, R. and Holmans, A. (1999), *Alternative Models of Care for Older People (With Respect to Old Age: Long-term Care – Rights and Responsibilities: A Report by the Royal Commission on Long-term Care, Research Volume 2)*, The Stationary Office, London.

Tollman, P., Guy, P., Altshuler, J., Flanagan, A. and Steiner, M. (2001), "A Revolution in R&D – How Genomics and Genetics are Transforming the Biopharmaceutical Industry," Boston Consulting Group, November.

UK Department of Health (2002), "Cost Effective Provision of Disease-Modifying Therapies for People with Multiple Sclerosis: Health Service Circular 2002/004", available at: *www.doh.gov.uk/ publications/coinh.html*.

UK National Auditors Office (2001), *Tackling Obesity in England: Report by the Comptroller and Auditor General*, HC 220, February 15, available at *www.nao.org.uk/publications/nao_reports/00-01/ 0001220es.pdf*.

US General Accounting Office (1994), *Cancer Survival: an International Comparison of Outcomes*, Government Printing Office, 1-45 (Publication No. GAO/PEMD-94-5), Washington DC.

US General Accounting Office (2003a), *Information Technology: Benefits Realized for Selected Health Care Functions*, Washington, October.

US General Accounting Office (2003b), *Nursing Home Quality: Prevalence of Serious Problems, While Declining, Reinforces Importance of Enhanced Oversight*, Washington.

Van Barnevald, R., Van Vliet, R.C. and Van De Ven, W.P. (2001), "Risk Sharing Between Competing Health Plans and Sponsors", *Health Affairs*, May/June.

Van Doorslaer, E., Masseria, C. *et al.* (2004), "Income-related Inequality in the Use of Medical Care in 21 OECD Countries", *Towards High-Performing Health Systems: Policy Studies*, OECD, Paris, forthcoming.

Whitten, P.S., Mair, F.S., Haycox, A., May, C.R., Williams, T.L. and Hellmich, S. (2002), "Systematic Review of Cost Effectiveness Studies of Telemedicine Interventions", *British Medical Journal*, Vol. 324, pp. 1434-1437.

Winslow, C.M., Kosecoff, J.B., Chassin, Kanouse, D.E. and Brook, R.H. (1988), "The Appropriateness of Performing Coronary Artery Bypass Surgery", *Journal of the American Medical Association* Vol. 260(4), pp. 505-509, July 22-29.

Wolf-Maier, K., Cooper, R.S., Kramer, H., Banegas, J.R., Giampaoli, S., Joffres, M.R., Poulter, N., Primastesta, P., Stegmayr, B. and Thamm, M. (2004), "Hypertension Treatment and Control in Five European Countries, Canada, and the United States", *Hypertension*, Vol. 43(10), January.

Wolfson, M. and Alavarez, M. (2002), "Towards Integrated and Coherent Health Information Systems for Performance Monitoring: The Canadian Experience", *Measuring Up: Improving Health System Performance in OECD Countries*, OECD, Paris.

Woolhandler, S., Campbell, T. and Himmelstein, D.U. (2003), "Costs of Health Care Administration in the United States and Canada", *New England Journal of Medicine*, Vol. 349(8), pp. 768-775, August.

World Bank (1999), *Curbing the Epidemic: Governments and the Economics of Tobacco Control*, Prabhat Jha (ed.).

PUBLICATIONS IN THE OECD HEALTH PROJECT SERIES

Towards High-performing Health Systems: Policy Studies (2004)

Private Health Insurance in OECD Countries (2004)

Health Technology and Decision Making (2004)

Long-term Care for Older People (2004)

OTHER RECENT OECD PUBLICATIONS

OECD Health Data 2004
(available in English, French, Spanish and German on CD-ROM (Windows 98, 2000, NT or Me)

Health at a Glance – OECD Indicators 2003
(published biennially)

A Disease-based Comparison of Health Systems: What is Best and at What Cost? (2003)

Measuring up: Improving Health Systems Performance in OECD Countries (2002)

OECD Reviews of Health Care Systems – Korea (2003)

Poverty and Health (2003)
(co-edited with the World Health Organization)

A System of Health Accounts (2000)

Measuring Expenditure on Health-related R&D (2001)

Genetic Testing: Policy issues for the New Millennium (2000)

Assessing Microbial Safety of Drinking Water: Improving Approaches and Methods (2003)

Xenotransplantation: International Policy Issues (1999)

For a full list of publications, consult the OECD On-Line Bookstore at *www.oecd.org*,
or write for a free written catalogue on Health to the following address:

OECD Publications Service
2, rue André-Pascal, 75775 PARIS CEDEX 16
or to the OECD distributor in your country

ALSO AVAILABLE

OECD Health Working Papers

Papers in this series can be found on the OECD website:
www.oecd.org/els/health/workingpapers

No. 15 **Private Health Insurance in OECD Countries: The Benefits and Costs for Individuals and Health Systems** (2004)

No. 14 **Income-related Inequality in the Use of Medical Care in 21 OECD Countries** (2004)

No. 13 **Dementia Care: A Comparative Analysis of Disease Management in Nine OECD Countries** (2004)

No. 12 **Private Health Insurance in France** (2004)

No. 11 **The Slovak Health Insurance System and the Potential Role for Private Health Insurance: Policy Challenges** (2004)

No. 10 **Private Health Insurance in Ireland. A Case Study** (2004)

No. 9 **Health Care Systems: Lessons from the Reform Experience** (2003)

No. 8 **Private Health Insurance in Australia. A Case Study** (2003)

No. 7 **Explaining Waiting-times Variations for Elective Surgery Across OECD Countries** (2003)

No. 6 **Tackling Excessive Waiting Times for Elective Surgery: A Comparison of Policies in 12 OECD Countries** (2003)

No. 5 **Stroke Care in OECD Countries: A Comparison of Treatment, Costs and Outcomes in 17 Countries** (2003)

No. 4 **Survey of Pharmacoeconomic Assessment Activity in Eleven Countries** (2003)

No. 3 **OECD Study of Cross-national Differences in the Treatment, Costs and Outcomes of Ischaemic Heart Disease** (2003)

No. 2 **Investment in Population Health in Five OECD Countries** (2003)

No. 1 **Pharmaceutical Use and Expenditure for Cardiovascular Disease and Stroke: A Study of 12 OECD Countries** (2003)

Other working papers also available from the OECD website include:

Labour Market and Social Policy Occasional Papers

No. 56 **An Assessment of the Performance of the Japanese Health Care System** (2001)

No. 53 **Towards More Choice in Social Protection? Individual Choice of Insurer in Basic Mandatory Health Insurance in Switzerland** (2001)

No. 47 **Performance Measurement and Performance Management in OECD Health Systems** (2001)

No. 46 **Exploring the Effects of Health Care on Mortality Across OECD Countries** (2000)

No. 44 **An Inventory of Health and Disability-related Surveys in OECD Countries** (2000)

No. 41 **Care Allowances for the Frail Elderly and their Impact on Women Care-Givers** (2000)

No. 40 **Pharmaceutical Policies in OECD Countries: Reconciling Social and Industrial Goals** (2000)

Health-related Reports from the OECD Directorate for Science, Technology and Industry

Digital Delivery of Health Care (2004)

Biotechnology and Healthy Ageing: Policy Implications of New Research (2003)

Genetic Inventions, Intellectual Property Rights and Licensing Practices (2003)

Biotechnology and Sustainability: the Fight against Infectious Diseases (2003)

OECD PUBLICATIONS, 2, rue André-Pascal, 75775 PARIS CEDEX 16
PRINTED IN FRANCE
(81 2004 08 1 P) ISBN 92-64-01555-8 – No. 53463 2004